T0122002

Esoteric Views on Health

A Medical and Metaphysical Look at Health Issues

Dr Hock Chye Yeoh
BSc, MBBS, DRM, FICGP, FIAMS, M.Med

iUniverse, Inc.
Bloomington

Esoteric Views on Health
A Medical and Metaphysical Look at Health Issues

iUniverse books may be ordered through booksellers or by contacting:

iUniverse
1663 Liberty Drive
Bloomington, IN 47403
www.iuniverse.com
1-800-Authors (1-800-288-4677)

Because of the dynamic nature of the Internet, any Web addresses or links contained in this book may have changed since publication and may no longer be valid. The views expressed in this work are solely those of the author and do not necessarily reflect the views of the publisher, and the publisher hereby disclaims any responsibility for them.

ISBN: 978-1-4502-6670-3 (sc)
ISBN: 978-1-4502-6671-0 (ebook)
ISBN: 978-1-4502-6672-7 (hc)

Printed in the United States of America

iUniverse rev. date: 11/11/2010

This book is dedicated to my parents for everything that they have done for me and my siblings. May the Heavens bless my father, Yeoh Khuan Wah, who taught us the Yang way and my mother, Nuah Gaik Kin (lovingly known as NGK) who gracefully showed us the Yin aspects.

Yin and Yang are the male and female qualities believed by the Tao. Interestingly enough we are of the Yang clan, if you know what I mean!

ABOUT THE AUTHOR

Dr. Hock Chye Yeoh is a medical doctor in private practice in Penang. He was very much a science orientated person until events in his life led him to search for answers and more meaning to an existence that felt incomplete. This exciting journey brought him to the world of esoteric science, meditation, feng shui, I Ching, Taoism, Hindu and Buddhist teachings.

In this book he describes his observations and imparts ideas he feels are extremely important. Most of his personal experiences are also described here, making this book very unique indeed as it blends science with the spiritual realms. Those patients who have been under his care and are open minded have certainly gained a lot from his insight. He is at the moment working on his second book.

ACKNOWLEDGEMENTS

I have many people to thank and among my first is the difficult to find Nadi Leaf reader, who interpreted what the saints and sages had written about me hundreds of years ago; perhaps even more than a thousand. The information that was revealed to me, mainly by St Augustine (354 – 430 AD) and by other Hindu sages gave me the courage to face my challenges and to return my karmic debts.

It was revealed to me that I should write a book and for many years I had no idea of what to write that would make a difference and fulfil a prophecy. Thank you saints and sages!

I must also thank a long time friend from Kuala Lumpur, Yap Siew Ying who introduced me to a world beyond scientific logic, turning me from a science nerd to a more balanced and open minded person.

The inspiration to write and the timing to do so, this I owe to my feng shui masters who taught me the secrets of the art and also to my unseen spiritual guides with whom I must have made contact through my meditations. It was through doing some feng shui calculations for myself that I realized it was the perfect time to write.

A big Thank you to my siblings Dr Hock Lye Yeoh, Milly and Annie Yeoh for they were eager to read the finished product as well as giving some very useful criticisms along the way. Some of my adventures were shared with them so many times and still they came back for more! Now they are repeated in print plus some other experiences I have never told them.

Special thanks goes to my wife, Melinda Koid, who would prod me gently to get me to work on this book whenever she caught me being a couch potato after enjoying the delicious meals that she always cooks.

A special mention to my beautiful daughter, Yen Theng, who is too young to read this book now but she inspires me everyday and for sure I will impart the knowledge to her.

I am deeply honoured and grateful to the family of the late Heng Hua Long for allowing me to narrate a story of the final days of Mr. Long, who played a significant part in my early years.

My next thanks goes to my Publishers for accepting this work and their staff who have given me much help along the way, in particular Eric Hanselmann.

My final thanks should go to my very capable editor, Sarah West. The manner of how I met her is an intriguing story in itself. I believe it was my spirit guides who led me to her. In fact the chapter on the Chakras was very much revised by her as it is her forte here. I believe she shares my visions for this book.

I wish to add that the author of the book 'Papillon', Henri Charriere, inspires me always by his reasoning that he had a better story to tell. I never forget that because I have the same feeling.

Finally it is best that I should acknowledge unseen helpers that have guided and given me the added inspiration to write.

Contents

ACKNOWLEDGEMENTS   vii
INTRODUCTION   xi
1.   My Journey   1
2.   Miss, you have Hypertension   14
3.   Something about Diabetes Mellitus   27
4.   Diagnosing Diabetes and Hypertension   33
5.   The Pitfalls of Treatment   38
6.   Obesity   42
7.   Re-emergence of Tuberculosis   48
8.   Cancer   53
9.   Dealing with Death   82
10. Supplements – Are they required?   97
11. A Guide to Supplements that make the Difference   104
12. The Tao of Chinese Medicine   119
13. The Chakras   126
14. Strange Illness caused by the Unknown   138
15. Meditation and Health   153
16. The Ultimate in Preventive Medicine   166
17. The Age of the Internet.   173
18. Coma, Dreams and Sleep   179
19. Big and Expensive is better…   192
20. Time to be a Vegetarian   199
21. Time to Discard Negative Attitudes   205
22. We Are All One   213
23. The Cosmic Man   225
Bibliography and recommended reading   228
RESOURCES   230

INTRODUCTION

This book is written with plenty of messages to all and I hope the contents will help many to understand the issues at hand and life in general. In my years as a medical person I have come across many incidents and issues that my wide variety of patients brought to my notice or that required my help. For those moments we experienced the same journey as co-creators and many a time it was my patients who taught me valuable lessons.

I had read many books and I thought it was time that I write one and make a contribution from my wide range of experiences. It is of no importance to me whether or not I become a famous author. What matters is if I can touch people's lives, increase awareness, give them hope, stir something within the hearts and minds of others and help make a difference. If one person is touched by my book and becomes awakened it will mean more than if many read it and feel nothing!

The topics discussed here have an extensive scope and are meant to provoke thought from the readers. I have kept detailed medical discussions to a minimum as I believe that with too much medical data and theory many readers may lose interest; besides this is not a medical text book.

I find, in my opinion that many health books deal with too many medical details which sometimes make up the bulk of the book or in an attempt to impress but could actually potentially bore lay readers and medically qualified people alike.

Many of the issues I write border around the philosophy of life, the esoteric pearls spoken from masters that I have come across or read through their works and my own thoughts. I touch on philosophy because if you understand the logic of my arguments, then you need not read medical texts nor say you missed medical schooling and wished that you had not. I strongly believe it is thus better to impart the philosophy and essence behind something rather than the great details of biochemistry, pharmacology and statistics which one will soon forget and the message is lost.

If you are able to understand the philosophy that I drive at you need not worry about the details, data and medical facts. I hope medical personnel will also read this book and gain a broader perspective that can work side by side with their medical training, for nothing is ever complete no matter how long we seek for answers and how much time is spent in any field of specialty.

I feel that the ancient civilizations of China, India and Egypt, among others have made several important contributions, many of which have been forgotten, rejected or neglected by modern day scientists. However, I draw much of my knowledge from the wise men of these ancient lands. The trouble with science is that it demands proof but many things can't be proven to be correct or to exist as yet, because science has not developed the technology or scientists reject these truths even when evidence is provided.

In my mind, these scientists are not behaving as 'real' scientists should. It is my opinion that some scientists are not open minded in certain areas and even when offered evidence, they will not believe it until they see it with their own eyes! Take the controversial topic of reincarnation. Much scientific verification has been collected on reincarnation by several renowned researchers, yet it isn't a well accepted idea to many spiritual people, let alone the scientists.

Even less demanding than the idea of reincarnation is the existence of ghosts and spirits and many do not believe that theses entities exist.

I was like one of those smart scientists - if you have no proof of something, don't even talk to me about it. But my life's journey made me do a 180 degree about turn. I now put my knowledge together in this book and present to you some of the things I believe no medical books even bring up in a single line not to mention a chapter. I offer both sides to each story, to show polarity - the negative and the positive so that you can put them together and form your own opinion. A whole new world awaits if you open your mind.

Dr Hock Chye Yeoh

1. My Journey

It is best to start with a glimpse of my own story on the journey of my life. When I was a small boy, I remembered that I was often sick and poor mum had to take me to see the government doctor. It was an ordeal to wait for the consultation and then for the medications. My frequent trips to the doctor made me wonder how he knew which sickness I had and what to give me to make me well. In other words I wanted to comprehend how a doctor thinks and diagnoses.

I needed to be one of them. Now that I am one, I realise that there are many things doctors know nothing about and what they do know, is not complete. This is despite the six long and strenuous years of toil and burning the mid-night candles, after which I embarked upon some specialized training to improve my skills and still it was not enough. I knew I had to seek knowledge elsewhere but I had no idea where.

Slowly my hard attitude was eroded by a very good friend who leant me some books to read. At that time, the only books I was interested in were medical journals of any kind. I felt that novels were totally a waste of time whereas factual books were more satisfactory. Though time was limited and precious, as any doctor will tell you, I started to read as many books as I could borrow from my friend.

The book that opened my mind was one on the magus of Strovolos, a wise man who could bilocate and heal illnesses that doctors had long since given up hope of finding a cure for and who wrote about reincarnation. It was not difficult for me to accept the idea of reincarnation basically because of my Asian values but to know that others from a different culture were thinking likewise was comforting.

This is what I meant by having deeper knowledge about life and searching for answers while my medical knowledge was only providing a very small part of the whole picture.

I had even for a time followed an Indian holy man and under gone Hindu rituals to cleanse myself. Years later, I made a pilgrimage to India to pay penance for a previous life episode. I travelled deep into the heart of India to complete my atonement and among the many things I had to do, one was quite funny. I had to travel to a Church in South India and just sit there after lighting candles for a full two hours! It was torture to me as this particular church was situated in a very remote fishing village and by the time I had reached it, I was really exhausted.

The other things I had to do were to feed the poor and at another village in remote Tamil Nadu, I had to pay respects and ask for forgiveness from seven ladies of the village. As I journeyed to give back all that I had owed, I began to understand more about my previous lives. I believe that my past existences were nothing to shout about and also I felt I must have been a terribly horrible person and thus in this lifetime I decided to turn over a new leaf.

Talking about leaves, I wish to include the 'leaf'' that changed my life. It was the Nadi Leaf. I had to track down the particular Leaf Reader, first in Singapore and then the trail led me to India.

Nadi leaves were written by Hindu sages hundreds of years ago, who after some deep meditation took on the monumental task of writing down prophecies of the individuals they were told to keep information on and who were not yet born. The name of the person and even their parents' names were recorded. These were written on leaves because it was before paper had been invented.

These leaves were stored in temples for safe keeping but some were lost or destroyed in the course of time due to termites, natural disasters, wars or theft.

The leaves that survived were distributed among the keepers of the leaves and thus they were spread all over India. You need to track down the correct keeper's descendants to be able to get your leaves read and interpreted and mind you India is a very large country. However I was led to the correct Leaf Reader by unseen hands although tracking him down was an adventure in itself.

After some years had passed I began the study of Feng Shui and took to it like a duck takes to water. I say this because deep inside me, I don't need any proof regarding the workings of this ancient Chinese art and science; somehow it just feels right and very comfortable.

Many years later, I found out the reason. I met a South African woman who is psychic and she would give me hints of my past lives. One of which was that I had been an advisor to an Emperor of China about architecture of the palace but died a disillusioned man when my advice was not taken. When I related this to a relative of mine with knowledge of Chinese history, he said that there was no one actually called an architect in old China but perhaps more appropriately they were known as Feng Shui masters!

I had to re-learn everything, having no memory of my past experience. I was lucky as various masters came into contact with me and I enrolled in their classes. It was one master who really "opened "my feng shui eyes and with his guidance I too gained the confidence of a master.

I also had the opportunity to be under one meditation teacher who teaches along the lines of Taoist practice but was only able to follow him at the most basic and rudimentary level.

Next, I took up Tai Chi to sustain good health and had the chance to learn it as an express student because I told the teacher that I was a busy government doctor and could not follow the slow snail's pace of learning the art. He was kind enough to oblige and I didn't disappoint him.

It was my youngest sister Annie, who introduced me to Reiki healing and persuaded me to go for it. My eyes were opened wider still and I began to see things differently.

I had also been very eager to know more about Buddhism and therefore enrolled for a diploma and was surprised that I could not attain the highest score and be the best student in class! It was indeed a humbling experience. I decided to expand my knowledge in Buddhism by reading more than just the books suggested in the course and began to understand why Albert Einstein, the Nobel Prize winner, had high regards for the Buddhist philosophy.

This was attributed to what Albert Einstein had said on Buddhism "Buddhism has the character of what would be expected in a cosmic religion for the future. It transcends a personal God, avoids dogmas and theology. It covers both natural and the spiritual and is based on a relative sense arising from the experience of all things natural and spiritual, as a meaningful unity."

I also accomplished a Certificate Class in Hinduism to compliment my Buddhist studies. My thirst for deeper knowledge in Hinduism started after I read the Mahabharata, Ramayana, Bhagavad Gita and the many books written by Paramahansa Yogananda. Again it was an inner peace-like feeling when I read these works and my soul did not reject any of the ideas, hence I took up serious studies in Hinduism. In my earlier years, I had followed a Hindu priest closely for several years.

My journey continued deeper along this path and I found myself being initiated into an Indonesian based religious order. The experience I had was out of this world.

The ceremonies I had gone through were simply magical. After an interview and screening by the "Bapak" I was allowed to be initiated into the order.

During the ceremony, I was surprised that my arms looked like the big scaly legs and sharp talons of an eagle; I even noticed feathers appearing on my upper arms. The master said he saw a huge peacock flying round the room during the initiation. I was told this was a good omen.

Another friend who was initiated a week earlier was disappointed in that his practice of the art was stagnating while I had good progress. It took me many years to appreciate the significance of the energy that arose in me as my knowledge grew and I was able to connect and combine what I had been taught through several modalities.

Many years later, I had to make the difficult decision of whether or not to be initiated into Taoism. I had under gone some purification processes and on the day of one of the initiation ceremonies I found myself in a group heading towards a temple, about 250 km away from where I live! This was despite being unsure whether or not to undergo the final ceremony. There was time to chicken out! Although I appeared calm on the outside, I was struggling within and had to keep reassuring myself with the knowledge that I could always change my mind.

We reached the temple by nightfall and my friend parked his car in the temple grounds and began to change into the attire for the ceremony. I had asked the Taoist gods for a clear sign to let me know whether I was making the correct decision. If I chose to take part and be initiated I would have to undergo a very strict regime for a complete year and I had doubts that I would be able to follow this discipline! Eventually I put on the ceremonial dress although I felt some reluctance having not yet seen any signs from the Gods to guide me in my decision.

I said to myself I could still back out at the last moment. This initiation process only occurs once in several years and through a very selective procedure, part of which was that we were to be recommended by our Grandmaster. We had to register our names and when I saw I was to be the 13th disciple that day I was full of happiness because that was the sign! You see, in our family, the number 13 turns out on very special and important matters! It is also a sign from my ancestors, giving their approval. This special number was recorded in our family history dating back several generations in ancient China. I was so pleased to be initiated. But there was another problem…

Being Malacca born, the land of the Babas of Malaysia I had very much difficulty in speaking the Chinese dialect which they used to converse. This was now the main worry. I told the temple officials and they assisted straight away with some coaching to help me answer some of the possible questions that our Spiritual Master would ask. He was to be channelled by the temple medium in a trance state. It was rather difficult to commit the phrases I learned to memory in such a short time and seemed even tougher than any medical exams I had sat!

The ceremony started and all of us had to attend a lecture by the Spiritual Master talking through the medium. Needless to say, I understood nothing, zero. Instead I tried to practice speaking in this unfamiliar dialect while sweating nervously at the same time. My only inner thoughts were 'Surely I will fail the question and answer time. Now what have I got myself into!'

Finally the moment arrived for the individual interview by Master. It was time to face the music and possible embarrassment. My heart was in palpitation. I had to carry a bowl of water in my hands and kneel down several feet away from Master, who looked so serene and dignified.

He asked me some questions, and to my utter and complete surprise, I spoke as if I knew the language – I was so fluent, the words just flew out of my mouth!

Master eventually pointed to my bowl of water and I saw, in a flash, a ray of light flew from his finger to my bowl, and I quickly drank the blessed water. Master then led us all in prayer to the Heavens and asked us to state our names out loud to the great Universe.

After the ceremony, I happened to take another look at the medium when he was out of the trance and noticed to my amazement, his face was totally different from the way he looked when he was in his state of reverie. I was quite taken aback. During the trance, the medium looked so dignified, like an emperor; his appearance also portrayed that of a wise man and with so much peace in his outlook. He spoke in a voice that was soft and yet authoritative. When the medium came out of his trance and mingled with us in breaking our strict vegetarian diet with a meal of fish and meat, to signify the end of the ceremony, I almost did not recognise him. He now looked so ordinary, like the 'boy next door' and spoke fast and in our local accent. The transformation was amazing!

This magical adventure named Taoism led me to the study of Lao Tzu's works and they were almost as difficult to understand as the I Ching which I studied some years later. It was only very recently however that I had a breakthrough with Lao Tzu's (born 600 BC) 'Tao Te Ching'. I needed to meditate while reading the passages and with the clarity that often comes with meditation, I began to understand at a higher level, the Tao of the Tao Te Ching.

It is the I Ching that still astounds me and keeps me spellbound. Somehow at that time I knew that I needed to embark upon and understand the I Ching and I thus began my search for a teacher. I had dabbled in it as an amateur and while I was working in London, I had tried to do some divination for a good Londoner friend.

He asked several questions on behalf of the various members of his family and I gladly did what I could at that time. Many years later, after I had left the UK, this friend managed to contact me and he informed me of astonishing incidents that had since come true for his family, especially for his only sister! She had taken my advice and never regretted it, saving her a lot of trouble! I was very surprised myself.

When I was working in Kuala Lumpur, a friend told me of a strange hermit who lived in the fringes of a small unnamed village at another very remote place, who knew a lot about I Ching and the Tao. I needed to meet this man and made arrangements with my friend to do so.

It took a long time to make the plans for the trip because the hermit had not wanted to meet anyone he didn't know, and strangely enough, especially anyone from the island of Penang, which is where I was residing!

I told my friend not to reveal this. From my persistent pestering, he finally agreed to try our luck and see if we would be able to meet the hermit without asking him first, as we felt for sure if we did his answer would be a 'no'.

We finally arrived at the hermit's very broken down tiny home, almost at the edge of the jungle. The door of the hut had some kind of deer antlers hanging on the outside and there were puddles of water in the immediate surroundings. Grass was over grown and other vegetation almost swallowed up the shabby wooden structure.

It was a perfect hideout I thought. However he wasn't in although the almost broken door was not locked. There was no need for security measures in such a remote place. So we waited outside for hours. Dusk was falling and then he appeared, looking extremely irritated at our presence but as he knew my friend, he attempted to restrain his annoyance.

He wore really old clothes but looked rather young and robust. My friend had a little conversation with him and finally the recluse turned to me and asked a few questions. We were now in his home and there was almost no furniture except an old bed and half a broken chair. The rest of the hut was filled with many kinds of dried herbs, leaves and some fresh jungle plants. The roof was full of holes through which the setting sun made a perfect natural light.

I waited for what felt an appropriate opportunity and took the courage to ask him if he would teach me the I Ching and the Tao. He answered me with a definite no! I tried my best to make him change his mind, giving several reasons - one was that it would be such a waste if he did not depart his deep knowledge on to someone.

He answered, "There is no worry - the Tao will never be lost; it always will appear to someone somewhere to carry on the knowledge."

Alas I knew this man would not budge from his position, I felt he saw me as an unworthy student. It was with great reluctance that I gave up and turned to other topics of conversation. Finally it was time to leave and he offered me some tea he had freshly brewed and we drank in silence.

Both of us were in deep thought. I then bade him farewell and we left but, not with heavy hearts, just meeting this man was in itself so exciting. Actually I believe he was right not to take me on as a student because it was unrealistic on my part - I was terribly busy working in the hospital, I would not have time to travel so far into the wilderness to spend more hours studying with him.

I later learned from my friend a little more about this hermit. Many years ago he was an engineer involved in numerous building projects and so knew a number of business people and government officials in the course of his work. It seemed that he knew a little too much about certain projects! This and his righteous ways made those involved rather uncomfortable. He was thus a misfit in that society and it was said that he had to flee for his life at one point after receiving various threats.

The years rolled by and after being on the run for several years, he finally found safety in the remote place we visited and settled down to a life of a recluse, edging a living by his herbal knowledge with plenty of time to meditate.

This story itself was being protected as no one knew his back ground in the place he had settled in. After I left his hut that day, I wasn't able to ever return as my friend made sure I would not remember the way there.

Many years passed and then a chance meeting with a metaphysical master from Hong Kong opened the door at last to my knowledge of the I Ching, so highly regarded by my feng shui Grandmaster.

While adding to my understanding of I Ching, I remembered many years ago I had bought a book in a second hand bookshop that includes the subjects of Feng shui and I Ching within its chapters. At the time I did not realize the importance of that book. I had somehow managed to find it in the bookshop amongst the mountains of old books and magazines which littered the shelves and were piled haphazardly from floor almost to the ceiling, filling every nook and cranny and spilling out into the corridors.

After buying this book which was later to become very important I put it away for safe keeping or perhaps a rainy day. When I dug the dusty old hardback out of my trunk and re-read it, my understanding of I Ching became greatly enhanced. It was as if a missing link had been filled which gave a sense of wholeness and enabled me more confidence in my calculations and interpretation.

I now know that I was guided to that shop and to the book, which suddenly caught my eye as I gazed in a daze at the heaps of books. In fact many of the great writings that I managed to buy seemed to beacon me in what I can only describe as a special attraction from the Divine! It seemed by chance I would drop into a book shop and be mysteriously drawn to a particular book ultimately proving to be exactly what I required to increase my knowledge and understanding of the esoteric.

A word about the I Ching - I had always respected the I Ching but its power needs to be experienced first hand to have an understanding of this great and multifaceted teaching of philosophical metaphysics; so very complex it needs to be taught by a master. One could read about it a hundred times and still not 'get' it. Even just to understand a little is considered a breakthrough. In my early days of experimenting with this extraordinary philosophy, I was literally being scolded by the I Ching for testing its patience with my repeated questioning and doubts. It was really very unnerving to be scolded by a book! This was conveyed by the trigrams generated during divination.

Not so long ago, having gained the necessary skill in using the I Ching, I had to consult it because my daughter was ill and she seemed not to be responding to all the medications I had given her. My wife was very worried and pushed my patience and confidence. I meditated and then used the I Ching oracle to seek an answer.

The message I gained from the I Ching was that I had nothing to fear as my daughter would recover. This was a great relief. What happened next helped to further reassure me and it must have shook the Heavens because my wife woke up in the middle of the night and with her own eyes saw Su Mu Kong, the Monkey God of Taoist belief. This great God was actually in our house walking towards our daughter's room to check or bless her! The very next morning her prolonged high fever broke and she had made a full recovery! This is one of the many miracles of alternative healing that doctors are unable to explain!

While my daughter seemed to be protected by the Monkey God, Su Mu Kong, I think I have an elephant spirit that guards me. Many years ago during my pilgrimage to the holy shrines of India, I saw a nicely sculptured wooden elephant that caught my attention. There were three such models but one was particularly attracting me. I had to purchase it and carted it along with me during my travels. I drew quite a crowd of curious on-lookers with my elephant I named Rajah.

When I took Rajah back with me to my house, I just decided that I should introduce Rajah to members of my family. So I carried Rajah and turned its face towards each family member, saying so and so is my relative who stays in this house. Then I put Rajah down, facing my front door and told him to guard the house.

That very night I had a dream of Rajah, he appeared as a huge, majestic bull elephant guarding my house, not letting anyone come in. He obeyed only me. People in the dream were frightened of Rajah.

Months later, when we were to perform prayers to my father, as we do yearly on the 7th moon of the Chinese calendar, I had another dream. In this dream, my father who had departed several years ago complained to me that Rajah did not allow him to even go near our house, so how on earth could he enjoy the offerings we had prepared for him.

The next morning, without hesitation, I took Rajah and held him facing a photo of my father, saying that he too was a member of our family though he had departed a long time ago. Since then, I never had any further complaints from my departed father.

Recently, I had to go for an over night trip to attend a medical conference and I told my little daughter to sleep in my room with her mother instead of her own room. The next morning the little one said she had a dream about a huge grey elephant looking at her. The elephant was not frightening to her as it appeared tame. I am sure it was Rajah checking on who was sleeping in my bed!

As you can see, my relationship with everything especially the I Ching is not academic but more spiritual and with a deep respect and reverence. To me, the I Ching is a living entity. Thus everyone's experience with it will be totally different, according to their level of being one with it.

Having gone through the various training modalities and studies, I realized that medicine is but so tiny a drop in the vast ocean of knowledge, truth and reality. Yet I see many medical colleagues of mine, whether my seniors or juniors, walking with an air of arrogance, as if they believe they know it all.

I do not regard my training in the various fields as nearly enough and I am constantly expanding my awareness. I am continuously refining myself as I make each little or quantum leap into higher consciousness. The difference must come from within and my outer world will change for the better. Even at this time, I am still undergoing lessons in a new system to prepare myself for the 'shifts' that will occur globally. I am learning to fine tune my vibrational energies, as the shamans of the Andes practised all those years ago.

I am so very thankful for every opportunity I have had to grow and I look forward with excitement and inner confidence to life's next adventure; feeling more prepared to journey into the great unknown. I am eager to paint my own picture on the blank canvas in front of me and leave my mark where once there was none.

2. Miss, you have Hypertension

Many of my patients get this diagnosis these days and most of them don't take it seriously. This is the typical reaction. They often say that they didn't get a good night's sleep, haven't been sleeping well lately; they were in a rush to see me or that this diagnosis was impossible, because just a few days ago they'd had their blood pressure taken by another doctor and it was found to be normal.

Some have even said that once they are on medication they will be stuck taking it for the rest of their lives or even worse - their neighbor alleged that taking medication would make matters even more severe and could induce getting other complications like kidney failure for example!

A new excuse to lie to oneself I heard the other day was 'But doc, I do lots of exercise, how could I possibly get hypertension?" Oh, if only life was that simple. I used to get very upset when they refused to believe me but not now. I am not here to save the world; you can always choose who to believe on medical facts, your doctor or your neighbors!

I let the Tao take its course. But when they come back with renal failure, heart attacks or strokes, what can I do? Only my best but even seeing the world's number one doctor may not reverse the damage to internal organs. It's bye-bye kidneys! Some will ask for public donations by appearing in the newspapers. Then kind hearted souls often make contributions not knowing it does nothing medically or karmically.

It never ceases to amaze me that most will believe their friends or neighbors and refuse further investigations and a re-check of their blood pressure by me. To this day, I have always wondered how their usual doctor would take their blood pressure readings and say they are normal.

It is little wonder that many hypertensive patients and/or diabetics end up with organ damage and renal failure requiring dialysis to survive. A poor quality of life becomes markedly reduced in lifespan not to mention the costs involved. This is a double or triple whammy and a life of regrets from the heart attack, stroke, blindness and heart failure that will certainly ensue if untreated.

Then, the direct selling agents of some multilevel marketing company will sell them very expensive products, "Here, take these, they will cure your pressure" but they have to keep buying the products until finally they go blind, have a heart attack or get a stroke! It's the same old story that I have heard so many times. Of course it's always easy to blame the doctor in the end, "You never told me, doc".

…And I will nearly fall off my chair!

This story was related by one of my nurses. Her relative who had been taking her hypertension medication diligently suddenly stopped the medicine because a neighbor warned her about the side effects of these tablets. Within a week they got news that she was admitted to intensive care after suffering a massive stroke.

The wise neighbor apparently had forgotten about the side effects of severe uncontrolled malignant hypertension. I call this the side–effects story. It seems that many folks are very clever about the down side of taking well trained physicians' prescribed medications. Let the Tao flow is what I say.

I really admire Lao Tzu and his Tao. In his day, which was nearly 2,500 years ago, he was so disillusioned with the politicians, the villagers and the rest of society that he decided to sit on his trusty buffalo and leave for the mountains never to be seen again.

In his book, on chapter 25, he said –

"There was something formless, yet complete
That existed before heaven and earth
Without sound, without substance
Dependant on nothing, unchanging
Its true name we do not know
Tao is the name that we gave it
Were I forced to say to what class of things
It belongs, I should call it Great
Now tao also means passing on,
And passing on means going Far Away
And going far away means returning "

To me this verse, as all the verses in his Tao, has such a profound message. But what intrigued me most was that 2,500 years ago, he faced the same human problems as we do today, perhaps the difference is the scale of negativity today.

Before going further, I wish to share the insight I have with regards to the Tao Te Ching which I had mentioned in the first chapter. For many years I could not understand the Tao and wasn't even able get a whiff of the message that Master Lao Tzu intended for us to know. This really troubled me very much for a long time. It was only by the method of meditation after each verse that I managed to get a tiny insight of his wisdom. And to prove it authentic to myself, I decided on a one sentence summary to test the power of understanding I had. Then it was another round of semi-meditation to comprehend this profound one sentence summary. It took me days to go through this process.

I found it hard to remember the important points raised by Lao Tzu and wanted a summary to help me utilize the ancient wisdom. Now, for the benefit of my readers, to save them time and frustration in deciphering the Tao, let me share with you my summary of part of his work.

Each numerical number comprises a whole chapter of the Tao Te Ching. To get a deeper meaning from each summary, you really need to think and ponder over each sentence to grasp the wisdom from it and in addition it is also advisable to read the original works.

Before I continue I would like to state that I believe if you do not understand yourself yet, you just can not understand the profound teachings of the Tao and I would not recommend you even think of the Tao without first understanding yourself to some extent.

1. The Tao, by not wanting to know it, you understand it.
2. All are One, in Unity and Harmony
3. Do not pursue material things
4. Tao is limitless, Abundance stays with the Tao
5. Do not discriminate; be impartial
6. The Feminine gives birth to the Creativity of Tao; Be a Co-Creator
7. Give without being asked and you attract everything
8. Be like water, go with the flow
9. Do not be greedy, where more becomes less
10. Have, but do not claim it all for yourselves; Have, but do not posses
11. There is a Centre for All things, yet it is unseen yet the most important
12. This World is an Illusion
13. Self itself is trouble; be above Self, be eternal
14. You are an Eternal Being having no form
15. Meditation has its benefits
16. Return to the Nameless and Placeless
17. Be the Enlightened leader who is actually invisible

18. You do not need rules to rule you; Have responsibility; be True Self
19. Be not attached to things - these are only forms
20. I may seem to be an idiot, but who is the Real Idiot? I get All from Source
21. Look no where else but deep inside you for the Tao!
22. Use the Law of Opposites to attain the desired
23. Nothing is constant, trust the Tao!
24. Destroy Ego
25. Understand This to know That
26. Above all, be calm
27. Truth is the Light and Great Teacher
28. If you preserve your Original nature, you can have every thing
29. There is a Time for every thing and Life is a movement towards Perfection
30. Success gained by waging wars will not last long. It is not the Way
31. War is not the Way - for Tao is of Life and Creation
32. All are of the Tao
33. Understand yourself, then only the Tao

I have stopped at the summary of Chapter 33 because as I was writing this paragraph, the message I received in my mind was that I am not doing justice to the Tao Te Ching if I summarise each great chapter in just one sentence. The book is so profound, it is difficult to read and figure out and I thought I was doing a fair job but when the voice came to me it stopped me in my tracks. I felt as though I was listening to the old master himself and I take these messages very seriously. One of the reasons for this is because many years ago, while experimenting with the I Ching, I knew I was being reprimanded and it was very daunting. It still seems to me now as though the I Ching is a living entity.

In fact one would definitely not regret treating the I Ching with the greatest of respect. Ever since that day, I have deep reverence for the

I Ching. Perhaps I will write another book just on the understanding of the Tao Te Ching but this will be a monumental task as many other authors have already done an excellent job.

To appreciate how complicated the Tao Te Ching is, I am reminded of the time Confucius had travelled a long way just to meet with Lao Tze. The two sages sparred, discussed and debated many points in their philosophies with each other and in the end Confucius had to admit that Lao Tze was a most complicated dragon.

Now back to the present day. I cannot blame the patients entirely for the choices they make as I feel it is up to us doctors to be aware of the latest studies and medications available. Some doctors never even bother to update themselves with new definitions of Hypertension or diabetes and treatment schedules etcetera. A number of doctors take no interest in their patients' welfare at all while others may do more damage rather than help cure or alleviate the plight of their patients. This is true of any other profession; it is a human ego problem and a huge one at that.

The ego is so damaging to one's progress in life if not checked or over come. I firmly believe it is the root cause of most problems in the world today as it was yesterday and as it will be tomorrow.

One of the secrets to a fulfilling life is to erase or delete the ego. The ego personality can manifest as hatred, jealousy, greed and many other negative emotions. A highly qualified doctor, for example may feel so important that he has no time to waste on lowly educated patients.

Even when patients are well educated, there are some doctors who feel the need to put them down one way or another, to show who is in command, thus leading to communication breakdowns and behaviour which is not in the best interest of the patient.

Medical science has progressed tremendously, there is no doubt. It has triumphed over many diseases and pathogens. However I feel it may have gone off track. Medical researchers have looked into the minute details of biochemistry, cell membranes and physiology even at the molecular level but I think they have missed the big picture.

This is because with each advancement in pharmacology at the molecular level by blocking receptors to modulate the pathology, the drugs went on to create other problems evident only after several years of usage by the populace. There are several examples like the Thalidomide story where severe deformations of newborns resulted; also in the COX inhibitors to treat arthritic pains but were thought to increase cardiac issues and so on.

In my mind, the yin-yang balance is of the utmost importance. These molecular receptors were there for a specific reason in the first place. To block their actions is to set an imbalance that will definitely result in another system being affected, hence the unwanted side effects of drugs at times. The yin-yang is the basic Taoist philosophy that has stood the test of time and is applicable to almost any situation.

Thus, if one really has hypertension, then a good physician may make the difference. The choice of drugs is of importance and several lifestyle changes need to be made. Many doctors just treat the hypertension but not the patients.

What I mean is that obesity needs to be dealt with, diet needs to be modified, bad habits curtailed and the patient should remain under the doctor's care. Some patients, upon being given the medication, will by-pass the doctor and buy the drugs on their own. This is not conducive as an expert opinion is still needed for follow up care; doses may need to be re-adjusted and blood chemistry determined. The DIY method just can not be applicable in medicine. A skilful doctor will use the right drug combination, which really does exist and enables safe and effective treatment.

Yet many have sought relief from herbal based products, thinking it is the better alternative. Herbal products once mass produced are actually no safer than any drugs. The catch word is "mass production"

– it is a manufacturing process and is still artificial in all aspects and suffers from the same profit centered thinking.

Most herbals have the concentrated active ingredients that make the herbs medicinal but once being so artificially concentrated as to have a faster effect, these active ingredients are no longer present in the specific ratios they consisted of in their native, original state – the state of yin-yang harmony of nature. This manufacturing process super imposes on the economics of profit making and the herbals become no different from pharmaceutical drugs. So, back to square one, and thousands of people are being led astray with the claims and hype of such industries.

Herbs in nature only produce a particular amount of the active principle under certain conditions, weather patterns and soil composition. These elements are stored in only specific parts of the plant. For example in some plants the active component is found only in the bark and not the leaves or roots therefore harvesting the leaves would be of no use in this case. Even collecting the bark where the active chemicals can be found is pointless if done all year round as the concentration differs in accordance with the seasons.

Bearing this in mind we find that herbal products manufactured incorrectly are no different from any pharmaceutical drugs in the final analysis. This is so often the case, although some can be found to have distinct advantages. It is the ones that make a difference that we are looking for and I have identified some and use them extensively in my practice with good results.

Diet plays an extremely important role in many diseases. The type of food intake now is all wrong – processed foodstuff is most detrimental to health with its preservatives, questionable quality of the food packaged and almost devoid of any vitamins. Likewise fast foods are fast lanes to ill health and obesity!

The increased meat intake is not on par with fresh vegetables and again the yin-yang balance is upset. Animals are fed with a variety of concoctions to hasten growth and we consume the chemicals within them along with the meat.

Do you know why we have Mad Cow Disease, which is fatal to cows and humans who consume the contaminated beef? The answer lies in the shocking fact that a group of cows were fed with ground meat based proteins and remember - cows are vegetarians! Man again was going against Nature and surely he will be punished.

When you break this natural Law what do you expect? Oh, but far worse, in my opinion, than the toxic chemicals given to these cows, are the emotions that all animals feel when they are slaughtered.

These emotions are stored in the muscles and as we consume the meat, we take in the negative emotional energies. That is why it is said that meat eaters have much anger and rage. The plant kingdom, with its lesser developed nervous system has less emotion stored and most vegetarians are more peace loving. Fishes are mid-way between animals and plants in the complexity of their nervous systems and thus do not cause that much emotional damage to consumers.

Those who are vegetarians may feel their minds more sharp and if they do meditation, their sensitivity will be increased and their powers of ESP as well. I know this because I was a vegetarian completely for a year once.

Humans are not all made equally, it was never meant to be and therefore every body has different requirements and people have to be treated as individuals. However it seems that on the whole humans were designed to be mostly vegetarian as their anatomy indirectly tells us with the molars and pre-molars to grind fibers and the longer intestines which are necessary for the digestion process in a vegetarian diet. Meat eaters of the animal kingdom have shorter intestines to quickly get rid of undigested food that can lead to toxins being built up.

Eating vegetables enables us to consume a wide variety of colors and to ensure a diversity of ingredients as each color has a different nutritional value and element. Our body requires seven colors just like a rainbow with the pot of gold at the end being our optimum health! Unfortunately due to commercial reasons, many vegetables are contaminated with chemicals to keep away pests and again we are back to square one. Organically grown vegetables are perhaps the answer but the higher costs make sure the masses can not afford them.

Exercise is an excellent way to keep a body healthy. However, the type of exercise is very important. The best forms are exercises such as brisk walking rather than the strenuous and joint jarring effects of jogging. In fact the very best forms of exercise are that of Qigong and Tai Chi. Do not be deceived by the slow movements of Tai Chi – it is really poetry in motion, when combined with the mind; a few rounds of Tai Chi is far more healthy than many rounds of jogging around the block. This is real exercise. Tai Chi is Yin, and Yin power is very great, as those who know Yin Feng Shui, the fengshui of graves, will attest to it.

The Chinese mind is hard to understand, their culture is even harder to comprehend. According to Taoist masters, qi flows where the mind concentrates, and slow exercises like Tai Chi allows the mind to control the flow of energy, the heart beat is not accelerated and thus maintains the longevity that is equated with a certain number of heart beats one is endowed with at birth – ie the lifespan. In strenuous exercise, you just have a faster heart rate that uses up your designated quota of heart beats. A friend of mine commented to me that after hearing my opinion on this matter he observed that most of his schoolmates who were active in sports are either now long dead or health wrecks!

I know many readers will say now this man is talking nonsense about a designated number of heart beats, what garbage! Well, I am not here to convince you of anything but only to share what I believe is truth. The choice of what to believe is always up to you along with the choice to have faith in the Great Masters and unseen forces at work first or wait for proof of their existence.

Anyway it is my belief that you have several lifetimes to make up your mind but as far as I am concerned this proof business is dangerous! Remember how some mathematicians can show you proof that 1 is equal to 2? Then they will put QED (Quite easily demonstrated) at the end of their proof. And now in the computer and digital age, you can cut and paste and create a photo of someone by combining his head to another's body and show this as verification. These are forms of trickery but there are also many more incidents where people wait so long for the proof of something that really does exist they miss out on all the benefits from it until sometimes it is too late.

That being said, however even the unseen energies of Qi Gong or Tai Chi may not bring down your malignant hypertension to desirable levels and you may still need oral anti-hypertensives. You still need the good old doctor.

This is not meant to be a medical text; therefore I shall not discuss further the various recommendations of expert committees on the types of drugs that are recommended as first choice in treatment regimes. Your doctor should know that or else sack him or her!

As far as Hypertension and Diabetes are concerned, the bottom line is don't waste your money on dubious products, don't waste your time on exercise only and don't waste your life by listening to neighbors and friends unless they are professors of Medicine or Endocrinology!

I think many readers would be disappointed with me in that I have not as yet revealed some secret remedy. There is simply none, it is plain and simple that these slow killers need the time tested medical drugs to just control the blood pressure or diabetes and not to cure it. There are at present no magic bullets to kill these vampires that come in the guise of hypertension or diabetes. You will need to find a dedicated physician who has your interest at heart. You will need to track him down.

This is what most doctors will tell you and what I believed myself to be the only truth many years ago. Now I do know of an essential ingredient, far more significant and without which even the best remedies will not work! Oh the remedies and doctors are very important but they do not work alone, Just as the yin needs the yang. I am talking about the power of the mind and positive thinking - about belief! We may need to see the right doctor and that we are taking the correct medication but we also need to believe it will work to see the results! Without a positive mind no amount of medicine is going to help you and yet when you take a leap of faith, what has taken years to accumulate as disease can be controlled, balanced, maintained and even cured in due course!

Nevertheless, science is progressing so fast now, that a medical cure may be available sooner than we think. Really, it is the slow way that hypertension and diabetes kills that is the most worrying part and without the power of the mind and awareness of the body those who have it will not see the enemy until it is just too late.

This is the hardest battle we doctors face, the slow and silent killers lurking around our patients who do not see the damage being done to their bodies slowly but surely. This is really what I want to emphasize, for if you know the enemy, you will know how to deal with it. This is Sun Tzu's Art of War (circa 500BC).

Another interesting detail I have observed is when a cure that is affordable to the masses is present, we find ourselves faced with some new or other chronic ailments to keep the yin-yang balance of human population and for the karma to manifest.

Then the scientist is back to square one again. Just like the game of snakes and ladders, where you get a long way up in the game and suddenly meet a snake and slide all the way back down again, such is life!

Just look at the example of antibiotic resistance developed by micro-organisms. Whenever a more powerful anti-biotic is developed to over come a bacterial infection soon the medication becomes less effective as tougher strains of the disease are produced to resist and overcome the medication and it becomes a vicious circle. This is also well seen in pesticides and in fact, in all the drugs and poisons that are developed. Surely we can take a hint from nature when we are faced with this 'proof' over and over again!

This is not The Way of the Tao. The hard way will always lose to the soft way, just like dripping water will erode the hard bedrock over time. Look at America, bombing the Viet Congs to kingdom come yet they lost the Vietnam War.

I myself have changed my strategy – I will always use the soft way to deal with my foes. I learned the soft way, the hard way! Perhaps this is why it is so meaningful to me. I think if we are all aware that there is an easier way it will bring hope as we realise that life is not meant to be a struggle but a stimulating journey with many clues and sign posts along the way! Life actually is to evolve to higher and higher levels. If you do not evolve but stay stagnant or worse still, retrograde, then you will be trapped in the Wheel of Karma.

3. Something about Diabetes Mellitus

As mentioned above, diabetes and hypertension share some similar points like being a silent assassin. That is why I will spend some time explaining about diabetes but without the boring details. If you wish to know more detailed information like the terminology doctor's use, then I would recommend a medical text book.

The International Diabetes Institute has recorded Malaysia as having the fourth highest number of diabetics in Asia with some 800,000 cases in 2007. These figures are expected to increase to 1.3 million by the end of 2010.

Diabetes is a worldwide pandemic, with 194 million or 5.1% being afflicted worldwide. About 75% of these will die of cardiac disease but with proper treatment with hypoglycemic (i.e. sugar lowering) agents all diabetic related deaths may be reduced by 42%. A decrease of 1% HBA1c could reduce the risk of diabetic complications by 21%.

The basic defect in diabetes is insulin lack, either from reduced production in the pancreas, defective insulin or receptor issues. The blood sugar is unable to enter into cells for their energy requirements and the cells are thus starved of nutrients, eventually some cells will die and among the first are the sensitive nerves.

It is a problem of starving in the midst of plenty. Just like so much money in the bank but it is not yours and thus you have no access to the account! You may even die of starvation. Oh, if you only have the correct ATM card (automatic teller machine) - insulin!

Again, what was written about in the Hypertension chapter can be applied here, it is the same scenario and the cycle continues. Those with both hypertension and diabetes suffer from double trouble where all complications are amplified. That is why doctors who realize this, need to be stricter in attaining acceptable levels of control. There should be no compromise or lackadaisical attitude from the doctor.

Poor diet has an even more direct effect on the cause of diabetes unlike in hypertension. The stress on the pancreas by the wrong intake of food will precipitate the onset of diabetes. With today's lifestyle, it is indeed small wonder why these metabolic diseases are on the rise. Poor eating habits include taking too much refined sugar, pastries and large carbohydrate meals with few or no vegetables required to retard quick absorption of glucose by the fibers in the vegetables and so on.

The latest reports from medical journals that even patients undergoing the best expert care, under strict scientific supervision, do not have blood sugar controls that are expected under these ideal settings are very worrying. These are experts and yet the results of blood sugar control are not as good as they ought to be. Now you can see that it is after all not that easy and the battle continues. This reason alone shows how important it is to have medical supervision and not to do it on your own.

There is even worse news - some studies managed to get almost perfect blood sugar controls and there is still evidence of micro vascular complications relentlessly marching on. Just think, if you are refusing to start treatment, then where do you stand? Many of my most educated patients still refuse treatment despite several counselling sessions and this is most disappointing. One more casualty to the disease will be claimed.

Now be prepared for a really out of this world theory of mine. I must warn that crazy as it seems, what I am going to suggest makes some kind of a sense if you consider it, if you think out of the box or what they call lateral thinking.

Now sugar is sweet, that is very basic and every one knows. It can be used to counter the bitter taste right? No need to think laterally here. But if we are so bitter about everything in life, in other words very frustrated and resentful, then this bitterness can only be countered by sweetness in the physical sense. Thus this could mean the onset of diabetes in such a person.

We live in a world of matter - dense matter at that. So diabetes, with so much sugar in the blood is a physical manifestation of a higher ethereal meaning. To change this bitterness in our mentality, we need to be more positive in our life. We need to stop the anger, the hatred and jealousy in our emotions. This is an important message from me!

It was the Chinese that first linked emotions with illness. Please refer to the Yellow Emperor's Book of Diseases or there is Louise L Hay's book entitled: 'You can heal your life.' Anyway, even if my mad theory is simply outrageous, but by simple logic, it is clear that positive emotions like happiness, joy, benevolence and kindness are a far better feeling to the person than being bitter every day, for their whole life.

A cheerful outlook in life will bring about more far reaching benefits than you can ever imagine. Really there is nothing to lose, well, only the negative things, if you follow my advice! In fact Taoists do Smiling Meditation; we smile at our internal organs one by one in this form of meditation, appreciating the work they do. This generates a lot of positive healing energy. In esoteric teachings from the East it is said that negative emotions attract negative entities and a happy, joyful person attracts the angels.

In reality I understand that, physical illness is first manifested in the non- physical bodies of man until it manifests physically in the body of matter. In our world of matter and time, it takes time for things to be crystallized. Thus real healing should take place in the levels of the mind, and surely but slowly will the body heal. Medical jargon merely describes the physical route and mechanism that is required for the physical world of genes, hereditary illness, DNA and so on. A thought comes first later translating to physical reality. This is the real basic working mechanism as understood by many masters.

The mind is not the brain. The mind has no physical attributes, it can not be grasped in the hand, but there is no doubt of its existence. The yogis, Buddhists and Taoists understand the mind better than many scientists who still tinker with physical matter. The physicists are the closest in understanding the phenomena of the Universe and they will be the ones who realize the wisdom of the Ancients. (Please refer to the Chapter 22 of this book for an in depth discussion.)

Many will protest to say that their minds and behaviour are neither that vengeful nor bitter and yet they suffer from diabetes. Well, one possibility is that for some, karma took a longer time to manifest and its appearance now is a sort of delayed re-action, the arrow finally landing on its mark. Perhaps for example a patient's leg was destined to be amputated made manifest by the diabetic condition.

The hypoglycemic attacks which diabetics sometimes experience may be an unexpected shock to new users of the oral medication. This can be a major setback in the fight against diabetes. The attacks which consist of cold sweats, shivering, feeling anxiety and tremors are enough to put patients off the medication forever. Their logic is "I was really feeling OK but since taking those drugs; I have had a bad reaction which made me feel terrible. Never again!" It is so damaging to the doctor's reputation and to the patient's well being in the long term.

Once it occurs, it is very hard to persuade the patient to continue with their treatment. Thus a skilful physician will make sure no such episodes occur or have the foresight to warn the patient. At least with some warning, the patient will feel less panicky should it occur and will know what to do.

The recent strategy of starting insulin analogues early in management to have better control may put many patients off, since it involves an injection. Again the technology is there but hampered by human behavior.

The very same advice can be given here as that offered to the oral anti-hypertensives – basically no magic bullets for a cure but plain and simple medications to control the disease and prevent all sorts of complications that will surely come if not under professional care. A small deviation here with regards to diabetes is possible though, as some Ayurvedic medications may work just as well as the drugs from the pharmaceutical industries.

Many doctors will notice that our population of diabetics and hypertensive patients are getting younger and younger, and so are cancer patients. Things tend to happen at an accelerated pace these days. Even heinous crimes are being committed by younger people. Like an 8 year old boy being found guilty of murdering his own mother. Again there are two ways to answer these phenomenons in our world of duality.

The most understood answer is that the lifestyle of today has changed to be more sedentary with computer games and the internet, the poor quality of modern processed foods and the stress in modern day living. The least understood reason requires much inner reflection, thought and perhaps meditation as it deals with the speeding up of karma, the Kali Yuga Age and Yin-Yang balance. These particular topics are not the main emphasis of this book. Esoteric knowledge is vast and I can only touch on the fringes of it to whet your appetite for you to discover your own truths.

I am a Truth seeker and am beginning to experience those feelings that indicate that something is absolutely right for me. I agree with what Buddha said, not to accept what he taught but to investigate for yourself and see and experience what is true for you. I cannot emphasise enough how experiencing truth for yourself is the most important teacher and how it helps you to reconnect with your inner guidance which is the most important advice pertaining only to you, that is available upon request at any time!

4. Diagnosing Diabetes and Hypertension

There are very few people who will go for a medical check up for fear of being told they have various problems. This is really the first stumbling block to good health and also the most difficult to over come.

The quality of the check up is yet another problem and I will discuss this later. The excuse of being too busy is a justification many use and is thus another foe against good health practices. Remember, every day can be busy and it is up to you to choose your priorities, we can always find the time to do the things we want to do!

Going to some private laboratory on your own is not recommended. You will need to visit your doctor who will get the correct type of blood screening to suit you personally and then should interpret the results accurately.

The many advertisements that lure the public to do blood tests by themselves are very damaging. The labs are mostly not concerned about quality and accuracy and will just toss the report to you without interpreting it. They are probably unable to do so due to limited knowledge mainly because they are not doctors.

Anyway they have collected your money and that is where their interest in you ends. I have seen this happening so often. Some are even far worse; their next step is to sell you expensive and dubious products simply because they are not allowed to prescribe the correct medication as they are, again, not doctors. Thus many are being fleeced for a second time.

I don't understand the logic of people who frequent these labs; it is like sending your car with a problem to a lawyer rather than to a motor mechanic. Even the best lawyer is unable to fix your car when compared with an average car mechanic.

There are many companies going to factories to conduct blood screening tests at a special package price but I feel that this is another way to rip off the innocent. I say this because many of my patients have paid even more and got far less tests done and the accuracy of the results were very suspect, making the entire exercise useless and money going into someone else's pocket. I will refuse to interpret these results as I don't know under what conditions the bloods were taken nor the accuracy of the laboratory involved.

The no time syndrome is also hurting many doctors themselves. They are so busy caring for their patients that they somehow forget about their own health. I have a surgeon friend of mine who was admitted to intensive care as suddenly he had chest discomfort and difficulty in breathing and was found to have a Blood Pressure reading of 180/110. He himself was very surprised at having such high blood pressure. Doctors are, after all humans too.

Medical check ups are no guarantee that all is well either. There have been cases I know of who have recently spent so much for a full medical but many months later had to be admitted to hospital for a stroke or even a heart attack.

There are two most probable reasons – one being the quality of the check up and secondly, inaccuracy or an error in the laboratory test results. Even under the best doctor and most accurate precise laboratory tests there is room for error and they are not always able to get the results 100% correct as one can in a mathematical equation. So I often tell my patients, nothing is 100% and Life is not so simple.

Diagnosing hypertension is easy but not always. I have a patient whose blood pressure is 120/80 which is normal but not in her case. This is because I had earlier records of her visits over the years and the readings were 90/ 70 when she first saw me years ago. Being well informed, or so she thought, she insisted that it was within normal range.

Another doctor who saw her confirmed her blood pressure to be 120/80 and reassured her that this is normal but the truth was in her case it wasn't normal at all. Second opinions sometimes do more harm than good, confusing the patient and complicating their management. There will always be those who seek a second opinion on a very clear cut diagnosis purely because they are not willing to accept the truth and will continue searching until they find someone who validates their opinion.

There is yet another enemy in the proper diagnosis of hypertension. Many medical personnel will advise the patient to come and take their blood pressure at least another four or five times just to confirm hypertension. Now this to me is a dirty trick most public hospital or clinic staff will use to get rid of the patient so that they will not be over loaded with work.

I have heard so many of my hypertensive patients complain that several years ago they were duly advised in this way and some shared that when they went for their blood pressure check, they had to wait hours just to see the doctor. Very often if doctors don't follow appointment times this also puts patients off from going as they often miss half a day of work sitting around waiting for what feels like ages. If for example, the patients are told to come at 9am but are kept waiting until 11 am, they may finally decide to stop going for the stupid follow up altogether and meanwhile their hypertension marches on.

Self diagnosis by patients is another problem we doctors face. Sometimes I hear of my patients having read some books or especially surfing the internet and coming to some fantastic conclusions that astound me! This is a perfect case then of how a little knowledge is dangerous and why I need not teach you how hypertension and diabetes are diagnosed, but would advise you to listen to your own doctor, who knows your case history.

As for me, I am giving you the esoteric philosophy to guide you from within. It is better to know that you have the ailment and to take positive action rather than being diagnosed with a stroke, heart attack, heart failure or renal failure.

Strokes are caused by either the rupture of blood vessels or emboli blocking the flow of blood to some region of the brain, resulting in partial or complete paralysis, as the ultimate in suffering from this condition. A stroke is the physical manifestation but the deeper meaning is much more. Again to some of you very scientific minds, what I am going to reveal may once again sound nonsensical to you but please keep an open mind.

Let us say for example that we have a person who is usually very busy, no time for anything, especially in the area of self care. There is no proper diet, he does not take care of his body which will have given him some signals if only he was in tune with it and so, to force his attention, the inevitable happens – a stroke!

This ensures that he will lie in bed and have the long awaited rest his body has been craving and gives him ample time for himself to reflect on his life thus far. He was living in the fast lane, so now he has had to slow down almost to a complete stop. All the pursuit of money and fame was after all not worth it, he now realizes. He had neglected not only his body but his family too. You may see this happening to people who lead very busy life styles with strenuous hobbies such as ski-ing, mountaineering or otherwise deeply involved in their business activities.

Now, having been compelled to stay at home to be with his family, it is not quality time, instead he needs their care and attention, putting a heavy strain on all resources. Many times our bodies would have communicated with us about something being wrong but either we ignore these messages or are totally impervious, unaware or unable to understand them.

I believe everything happens for a reason, which is of a higher nature but to be manifested in this world, a physical sign ensues. This world is a world of Maya, of Illusions, as Buddhists know it. Just look around you – illusions are every where. The rich man, do you think he is happy? It is just an illusion that he is, for he may have investments that are draining his reserves and causing him to be worried sick.

The beautiful woman, do you think she is happy? She is probably anxious about the onset of and how to cope with old age that no mortal escapes.

The fear of being diagnosed with Hypertension and Diabetes have kept many who suffer from it away from the doctor and this is certainly not the way to deal with a silent, slow killer. You must know your enemy as Sun Tzu wrote in his military strategy manual.

After the initial shock of being told one has either Hypertension and/or Diabetes, I will tell my patients to look on the bright side as now we can initiate remedial measures to stop or at least retard the micro and macro-vascular complications. Otherwise to remain undiagnosed for a few more years will lead to very unfavorable results as far as their health is concerned. I always like to give my patients hope and uplift their spirits to ensure a positive outlook and therefore optimum results.

5. The Pitfalls of Treatment

There are very effective medications to deal with hypertension and diabetes. The problem is patient compliance to the medication. Some are very smart, they will take the medication on alternate days, thinking by doing so they will reduce the side effects they have heard so much about from their friends or from their research.

This alternate day regime does more damage than they think. First, it does nothing to control the disease; the erratic control on the whole is no control at all when averaged out and gives both patient and doctor a false sense of security. It is as though no medication is given and the relentless march of the disease continues.

Others fool their doctors and themselves really, by only taking medications a few days before their clinic appointments to deceive the doctors into thinking that they are compliant with their medications and show that the blood pressure or diabetes is under control. If the doctor is on the ball these patients can still be helped. This takes a doctor who understands and is willing to go deeper and counsel those who obviously very much need compassionate care.

The worst are those who disappear from follow ups and we think to ourselves - God knows what has happened to them. Most of such patients end up with the most feared of end stage complications. Then all their running to the best hospitals to see the finest doctors will come to nothing - zero. It is too late. Oh, I see so much of this example. This story keeps repeating in a never ending cycle, so it seems.

My strong feeling is that the charlatans who have been 'treating' these people have blood on their hands, it's as simple as that. What heavy karma they bear. I am referring to those who sell them products that are of no use, or who give wrong advice, medically or otherwise. This includes doctors and related health personnel who are not taking good, professional care of their patients.

In fact, I grade this type of crime as among the worst, for they should know better. As I have always said to my friends, if there is such a place as hell and we are able to take a peep inside, we would certainly find plenty of doctors, lawyers, engineers, politicians, pharmacists and so on because of the great sins committed by some of them towards society through their greed and irresponsibility!

Some doctors like to use the latest drug in the market but I am not one of these trendy types because invariably some kind of reaction will surface after widespread usage. Besides, these state of the art drugs are not cheap and defeat the purpose of helping patients who need to use long term medication and be able to afford the ongoing costs. It is best to stick with affordable drugs that have been around for a long time and with a clean track record as at the end of the day, blood Pressure and good blood sugar control are the most important issues.

Many doctors are too drug crazy but forget about important issues such as a patient's weight reduction in relevant cases. Reducing weight will go a long way in controlling a diabetic patient's condition and with the correct food intake and recommended exercise regime perhaps some may not even require any medication at all.

It is not necessary for me to write which drugs are needed for the treatment of these chronic diseases as it is not the purpose of this work. The drugs needed should already be in the arsenal of any good doctor.

There are medication related issues of course and certain drugs do cause more problems than others and therefore it is of utmost importance that doctors are aware. Some are very expensive as mentioned above and it is of value to know which medications are less costly but just as good as the latest and most expensive ones in the market.

After seeking a dedicated doctor who knows his stuff, the main problem is again the patients themselves - will they keep their part of the bargain and be compliant both with the medications and the guidance given by the doctor?

Although I am talking mainly about the treatment of diabetes and hypertension, the advice I have offered above is the same for the treatment of all diseases or issues requiring the taking of medications of any sort.

To give an example of how important it is to be discerning and not influenced by experts pushing their brand of drugs I once attended a medical meeting on the latest of the oral contraceptives that were being introduced to the world.

There was a professor from Chicago doing the presentation and answering many scientific questions from an audience of medical professionals.

After the session, I was having a cup of coffee by myself while most of the doctors were leaving the place. The drug representative, a lady, came up to me for a short chat and asked me the forbidden question – how I felt about their new product. I asked her if she would accept some hard answers from me and she said, 'Shoot, doc." So I shot!

I told her that there are some developed countries in the West and countries like Japan and Singapore which do not require a new contraception as their populations are actually dwindling due to the fertility rates ever decreasing.

Countries with booming populations and high fertility rates may need these contraceptives but they will probably not be able to afford them. To me it made no sense and the scientists were just wasting their time. Thus I told her I will not use their product. End of discussion! …And chapter!

6. Obesity

This topic needs to be included as obesity is becoming an almost world wide epidemic. Countries like Singapore, Malaysia and China are not spared.

The flourishing of slimming centers is an indication of the neglect from the medical community to see how important it is to treat obesity and curb this problem before it even starts. This is a shame indeed as people fall prey to these centers that provide at times very dubious methods of reducing weight and on the very top of this are the exorbitant fees they charge.

There are cases where the surgical methods used have resulted in death of patients, despite the surgery being conducted by experienced and qualified medical doctors. In the UK, every year the surgeries have resulted in 30,000 obesity related deaths and 18 million days off work due to obesity related medical ailments.

Children in several countries are getting obese at a younger age which further compounds the issue.

A healthy body mass index is between 20 – 25 BMI (weight kg/height m2), being over weight is 25 – 30 BMI, being considered fat being 30 – 40 BMI and the label obese is for those over 40 BMI. It is a serious health issue to be at this weight. Apart from not looking like a model, the real issues are the health risks associated with obesity. The summary of the health issues secondary to obesity can be seen below.

Greatly increased Risk of – Diabetes

    Hypertension
    Dyslipidaemia
    Breathlessness
    Sleep apnea
    Gall Bladder disease

Moderately increased Risk of – Coronary heart disease

    Osteoarthritis
    Gout
    Pregnancy complications

Increased Risk of – Cancers

    Impaired fertility/ Polycystic ovarian syndrome
    Low back pain
    Anaesthetic risks
    Fetal defects
    Stroke
    Cataracts
    Pancreatitis
    Skin disorders

GYNAECOLOGICAL COMPLICATIONS

    Promotes ovarian androgen secretion (hirsute, acne, alopecia)
    Dysfunctional ovaries
    Venous thrombosis

OBSTETRICAL COMPLICATIONS

Infertility
Miscarriage, fetal abnormalities
Pregnancy induced Hypertension, PET, Gestational Diabetes
Shoulder dystocia, caesarean section
Post partum hemorrhage, Thromboembolism

OTHER PROBLEMS ENCOUNTERED

Difficult ultrasonography
Large BP cuffs needed
Reduced awareness of fetal movements
Difficult electronic fetal monitoring
Anesthetic risks
Wound care compromised

From the list above it shows how important it is that we attain normal body weight to experience all its advantages. These are –

The Blood Pressure falls
Blood glucose levels fall by as much as 50%
30% increase in insulin sensitivity
40 – 60% fall in incidence of diabetes
10% fall in cholesterol
30% fall in triglycerides
30% fall in all mortality caused by disease
30% fall in deaths related to diabetes
40% fall in deaths related to obesity alone

I remember a terrible experience I had with an obese patient who had appendicitis. The operation itself was technically difficult due to the size and layers of fat. Post operatively all was well and he was about to be discharged when he suddenly died from cardiac arrest. I was badly shaken and took a week to regain my self confidence to go to the operating theater again. Obese individuals have a severe risk of post-operative complications, even the so called safer liposuction. This simple procedure has already claimed several lives.

There are so many methods available to lose fat but in reality, almost none will result in a permanent state. Unfortunately this is more real than anyone cares to believe. No matter what method you try, the fat will return slowly but surely until the basic cause has been addressed in almost all cases. Even if all medical causes were ruled out by a thorough investigation plus the fact that the person swears that he or she eats very little, then there is still a hidden cause which is esoteric in nature. However, let me deal with some causes that I have noticed in many of my patients but have never seen documented anywhere.

I observed that those who swallow their food without chewing properly tend to gain weight. The only reason I could think of is that with improperly digested food, less nutrients are being absorbed and thus the body needs more, and yet is almost never fulfilled. The vicious cycle continues and weight is being gained. Many try to lose weight by cutting down their food intake to one meal a day. It works for some but for others, it stimulates the body to store energy as it interprets that there will be a coming famine and it is better to make hay while the sun shines (i.e.: store more fat).

For this group of individuals, they must eat small meals three times a day. The majority however consumes just too much food in all forms and yet they do not think of it as over indulgence. There are no fat people in the land of famine is what I always tell these people who gobble food like there is no tomorrow!

There are actually only two types of pills approved for weight loss – Orlistat and Sibutramine, any other medications are not safe and are actually illegal. Even these two are not my cup of tea, as they prove to be troublesome as well. The really obese patients need more drastic measures and surgery is what doctors can offer. There are various types –

- Roux- en-Y gastric bypass

- Gastric banding
- Biliopancreatic diversion with sleeve resection

Surgery, of any type, is always risky with several possible complications like:-

- thromboembolism
- bleeding
- pneumonia
- stenosis
- ulcers
- peritonitis
- iron deficiency
- calcium and vit. D deficiency
- vit. B deficiency
- protein deficiency
- gallstones
- death (1%)

As you can see it is really an exchange of problems rather than a solution. The answer is not more drugs or more types of sophisticated surgical methods. A healthy diet seems a much better choice and thus I recommend to my patients a special mixture of 'super oats' that a friend and I worked on and formulated. They seem to do a good job, especially when consumed in combination with our fiber which is another of our uniquely formulated products.

Still we can not claim complete success because there is a category of obese individuals whose obesity I believe, is brought from previous lives. They had not learned to overcome their obesity in any life and so it keeps repeating in every reincarnation.

Others try to use the wall of fat to insulate themselves against the outside world. Here I am talking about deep secrets that even the individuals will not be aware of themselves. Some use this wall to protect themselves from the outside especially in the case of women who have been abused by men; they use fat to make them socially unattractive so that they will not attract another man into their lives.

There is also a large group of people who are sad and lonely or feel something missing from their lives and they use food as comfort. It becomes their friend and temporarily fills the void. In these categories, no amount of surgery, medication, exercise or diet will bring an end to their problems unless their higher Selves want to stop being obese.

Some souls are comfortable with a big, round body and they keep this shape reincarnation after reincarnation. However the majority are just leading a bad lifestyle in this modern era with rich fatty and sugary foods and little exercise, it is pure and simply just plain, laziness and greed.

Now that you know what the dangers of being overweight or obese are, it is time to take action either proactive or reactive. For those of you who are overweight do not give the excuse that your body weight is due to previous life issues - how do you know?

I believe the ultimate solution to obesity is self worth. When you love yourself you will be attracted to all things good for you and this is the easiest way to flow with the chi towards a healthy lifestyle, naturally and without struggle.

7.   Re-emergence of Tuberculosis

I did not think I would be including this chapter in a modern day setting but things are getting almost out of hand with Tuberculosis the world over. In bringing this topic out here, I hope to warn the public and doctors as well, to be more vigilant in this new emerging threat from an old foe. At the time of writing, it is believed that one third of the world's population is infected with this TB bacillus.

In 2005, the largest number of new cases occurred in South East Asia. The figure for 2008 in Malaysia was 16,325 cases of TB, of which 2,050 were foreign workers, which was 36% of all foreign workers in the country.

It was second only to reported Dengue cases, which stood at 17,047. The bacterium was first identified in 1882 and has now evolved to a new strain that is resistant to many drugs, now referred to as MDR TB, multiple drug resistant TB. This strain is resistant to what used to be the most effective drugs, Isoniazid and Rifampicin as well as one of the three injectable second-line drugs like Amikacin, Kanamycin or Capreomycin.

This dilemma therefore leaves doctors with very little alternative drug treatment to combat the disease. The situation is compounded by the spread in HIV patients. TB is often the cause of death in these patients before they reach full blown AIDS. It seems they have to deal with two enemies and it is double trouble for this group of vulnerable patients whose immunity is already being compromised.

For Malaysia, in 2008, there was a reported 63.1 cases of TB per a 100,000 population, putting the country as an "Intermediate Burden Country".

About 10% are also infected with HIV. The situation is made worse by the immigrant workers from neighboring countries that carry the infection despite the screening methods already in place.

At the time of writing, in Chicago, USA, it was reported a trainee doctor working in the paediatric wards of a Chicago hospital was diagnosed with TB and had in the course of his work, exposed about 80 babies and 140 co-workers to the TB bacilli, which is spread by droplet infection from a cough, sneeze or even normal talking.

Areas that have been exposed to the infection and are closed in with little or no ventilation increase the risk of catching diseases such as this. Public places like cinemas, halls, pubs and public transportation such as trains, buses and planes are thus the most likely places for infections to spread.

Any cough lasting more than 3 weeks after taking the appropriate medication warrants a screen for TB especially if this is accompanied by low grade fever at night, loss of appetite and weight.

Sometimes there can be atypical presentation of symptoms which could lead both patient and doctors off track. The message here is never treat a so called simple cough yourself with over the counter medication at the drug store or by a pharmacist. Seek a proper medical opinion.

Do not take a cough lightly. Chronic coughs may also mean another sinister problem – that of lung cancers. Here I wish to high light a case of my own cousin, Eng. She was married to a man from a poor family and to save costs, sought treatment of her long standing cough from the many pharmacists around. However the cough persisted. Finally, out of desperation, she consulted me.

To my horror, I discovered that she had ovarian cancer and I referred her to our public hospital, as they could not afford private care. The doctors there operated on her only to find an inoperable tumor and then subjected her to an intensive regime of chemotherapy.

However, from that instant onwards, she went down hill and was warded in the intensive care unit. Even with my heavy schedule, I visited her to give moral support, always giving her positive encouragement until her last day. She was only 43 years old. If only she had consulted me much earlier, a better outcome would have been possible.

Now back to the bacteria. You can see that the world need not require new unknown bacteria or viruses to cause an epidemic - our old enemies that we thought were beaten by modern medicine have come back to haunt us with a vengeance.

Yes, even lowly forms of life like these bugs evolve through the course of time to out wit us. So who is smarter? Many research scientists in the medical circle take pride in their evidence based medicine these days. However, I have always smiled at this magic word among doctors because I knew it was all basically nonsense.

For those who are new to this term evidence based medicine, let me enlighten or entertain you a bit. At every medical conference nowadays they talk of evidence based medicine or EBM. EBM is the integration of clinical expertise, patient values, and the best evidence found in clinical research used in the decision making process for patient care. Looks great theoretically but practically speaking, the evidence can be tainted.

One case is so embarrassing for the medical community. The following results were reported in a randomized controlled scientific trial. It was noted that the use of the perioperative beta-blocker Bisoprolol in patients undergoing major vascular surgery caused a 100% reduction in the risk of non-fatal myocardial infarction and an 80% reduction in the risk of cardiac death.

Due to this very important and significant life saving result, the trial was stopped quickly in order to have the information reported in medical journals as soon as possible. This was evidence based and many doctors applied it blindly. However it was later discovered by another scientific investigation that the reduction in myocardial infarction was only 27%. More importantly, there was a doubling in the risk of disabling strokes and a 30% increase in the risk of death. So the 'evidence' these brainy scientists are talking about in evidence based medicine is often inconclusive.

Usually when research studies are conducted people focus and attract what they want to hear. This is why you can have many studies on one subject with various results. It is up to us doctors to look at all scenarios and make an informed opinion and not follow these guidelines blindly. However it is still essential that the scientists at the forefront of research look closely through the microscope at their own work before introducing their theories to the world.

I continue to read medical journals to keep myself abreast but somehow I can also see the forest for the trees, meaning I can see the bigger picture and smell the scientific flaw of focusing on one tree when there are many others in the forest. I just smile to myself and discard the evidence based medical break through when I spot such a flaw.

Sadly, many doctors will stick to what the journals print without using their own rational minds. Partly because they have not done research work and do not understand the fine print in terms of statistics and the research methodology. I participated in many such activities while based in London and it opened my eyes as to the research process. So far, the battle with the tubercle bacteria goes on with Mankind losing ground at the moment.

According to TCM (Traditional Chinese Medicine) principles, the lungs belong to the metal element, which is controlled by the heart and is one of the zhang organs. The emotion that can damage the lungs is grief and according to its severity, can manifest as lung disease or cancer.

Tuberculosis was known as consumption in the old days and now you may see the link – if one is greatly consumed by grief, lung diseases can manifest. It is most interesting to see how clever the Universe is with its languages full of deeper meanings such as this to help guide us at every turn.

To conclude I would say take care of your body. If you feel a cough or cold coming on or if you already have respiratory problems then foods that are of cold constitution e.g.: miso, spinach, coconut, mushroom should be avoided to protect the lungs; whereas food like wheat, lamb, garlic and onions are recommended to strengthen them.

An old foe is re-emerging and all of us must be vigilant in being aware and listening to the messages our bodies continually express. If you learn to be in touch with all your senses you will 'feel' what the body requires to be healthy.

8.   Cancer

All countries are not spared from this dreaded disease and in Malaysia, which is expected to reach a developed country status in 2020 it has already reached a very developed country status as far as heart disease, renal failure and cancers are concerned. About 13.8 per 100,000 population are likely to have cancer of the bowel each year which works out to be about 3,900 new cases in a year in a population of 28 million. This comprises of about 14.5% of all cases of cancers reported among males in 2005 and about 9.9% in women.

Not everyone will experience the problem yet when it occurs; it has far reaching consequences for the patient and close family members. Unless one's own family member is affected, many do not grasp the devastating effects cancers have on the entire family.

Apart from fear and worry, unfortunately the bottom line is money, as the treatment is costly. When a family member is first diagnosed, everyone will want to get the best care for their loved one. The costs involved can be staggering and quite a few would have to turn down state of the art medical treatment due to these high costs, especially if they have no insurance coverage.

Many will try to do their best and everything possible for the family member concerned and pool their resources but the battle with cancer can be long and I know of many families being exhausted financially by six months and the repercussions will linger even longer. Savings can be depleted and credit cards used to the maximum.

Some end up selling their properties, jewellery or borrowing from close friends and relatives and then resort to loan sharks. If they are lucky, it will take them a few years to recover from the financial disaster apart from losing their loved one in spite of all the heroic efforts both by the doctors, specialists and themselves.

A large number will need to go to public hospitals run by the government but the waiting list can be so long, even for an MRI scan not to mention radiation therapy or other treatment modalities and many are forced to seek private hospitals to save time in waiting for an appointment. That is when the nightmare starts.

There are also many hidden costs which many do not realize, these include transportation, food supplements, non-prescription medicines, nursing aid or maid expenses, telephone bills and complimentary medications and the lists go on.

Family squabbles often arise because some will not chip in nor give moral support. Things can get to be really complicated and very ugly when personal issues are brought up from the past. All of these tend to surface and test the family. Thus one case of cancer may bring down an entire family – draining them emotionally, financially and physically.

Now everyone has heard of the devastating effects of cancers and perhaps equally horrible are the modes of treatment. Let me start with cancer of the lungs in a serious medical manner. Lung cancer is divided into small cell type and non-small cell type, the latter makes up 90% of cases.

The small cell type remains deadly and very aggressive, with most patients dying within 2 years. The non-small cell is divided into early operable and the late stage non-operable types. This late type is further divided into squamous and non-squamous types. Treatment for non-squamous is pemetrexed. Other effective drugs can be cisplatin, carboplatin, gemcitabine, docetaxel, paclitaxel, vinorelbine, bevacizumab, cetuximab, gefitinib and erlotinib. The drug gefitinib works best for cases that have the EGFR mutations.

I have limited technical data to a minimum but feel that due to the severity of this issue it is important to go into some specifics. Of course oncologists will be in a better position than I to talk further.

It makes me wonder, and others who think alike, why with all the medical advancements in oncology, chemotherapy, radiotherapy and surgery, we still have dismal survival rates. To be fair, there are very good survival rates for early stage cancers and even some advanced ones, yet over all, the picture is not acceptable.

The very good rates of survival are from the best hospitals with world renowned specialists but most ordinary cancer patients are from places where such good expertise and facilities are not available. It is thus in my opinion, not relevant to talk about these survival rates as it does not apply to many. Even those with the best rates are actually misleading, as they are only talking of 5 year survival rates. This is simply because there is no cure as yet. A bold statement came from Allen Levin MD, who wrote in his book "The Healing of cancer" published by Marcus Books, 1990 – " The majority of the cancer patients in this country die because of chemotherapy, which does not cure breast, colon or lung cancers. This has been documented for over a decade and nevertheless doctors still utilize chemotherapy to fight these cancers."

This could only mean that research is on the wrong track. The targets are the cancer cells and the goal is to kill them but in the process many normal cells are affected and this is the severe side effect of chemotherapy.

No matter how specific the chemotherapy agents are, still a population of normal cells are likely to be destroyed. To me, a completely new mode of treatment needs to be devised; otherwise we will be stuck at square one for a long time to come.

I believe the approach of the pharmaceutical industry is wrong as whatever drug they discover now or in the future, is quite a waste of time and money. Although the new drugs will be more potent and specific, the same old issues remain – no cure but instead more problems being created.

In the 2009 publication of Archive of Internal Medicine, it was reported that in the largest study involving more than 161,000 post menopausal women, multivitamins do not prevent cancer or heart diseases. So what can many say about this? The answer is apparent when we discuss more in the passages that follow.

Many who suffer from cancers ask the question why they get it. Medical science may give part of the story only. The toxic environment, chemicals in our food, depressed or ineffective immune system, hereditary genes, mutated genes or even just de novo. Many more causes may even be discovered especially new types of viruses. Whatever the cause may be, those described are the physical causes. I think part of the real issue is something that can't be seen or quantified.

As long as we look for physical causes, we will miss the real issue. Yes, another chemical identified as a carcinogen will be discovered, but this does not tell the whole truth or picture. Beyond matter is the Mind. The mind is very powerful, and just the fear of getting cancer may lead to cancer manifesting. Behind the mind, there is something more fundamental; some will say it is fate, written in the stars. This is only partly true and we need to go way beyond as now we are only scratching the surface.

I believe the Buddhists are close to getting the answers and I am referring to bad karmic manifestation. We reap the seeds we sow, with this; we can have a single theory to explain all types of cancer occurrence.

The bad karma needs to be manifested in this particular life time, and thus the physical conditions are met to allow for the physical appearance of the cancer to manifest. Thus, the person who may have been very kind hearted, and a pure vegetarian too, could still get cancer due to the karma of past deeds. It is pay back time.

Sometimes there is no bad karma to cause the cancer, but the soul agreed to have cancer in the physical body so as to experience pain and tragedy, to teach a lesson to the people whose lives are entwined with theirs.

So the person may under go all types of treatment for which there is no cure because the soul is determined to go along with this suffering to fulfil a higher divine plan. If the lessons have been learned in some other way this could explain the soul's decision not to continue with the suffering and will explain why some cancer patients have spontaneous remission or disappearance of the cancer.

I feel that those who do not believe in past lives, reincarnation and karmic debts may want to take a very good look at this topic at one time in their lives. If it is not mentioned in your belief system it does not mean it doesn't exist or hold true. Anyway, the karmic angle will explain beautifully many situations.

The karmic theory can explain why someone can smoke heavily and not have lung cancer while a non-smoker is mysteriously afflicted with the disease. The same goes for why cancer would affect someone who is very careful with their diet, or why some feng shui masters attribute getting cancer to the bad house feng shui, be it of the flying stars or landform schools of feng shui. As I do feng shui audits for some of my clients, it is uncanny that some people are simply blessed with houses that have good feng shui while others, look high and low for such houses and can not find one.

I remember a case I had. This family was in a desperate situation – financially as well as in health issues. The feng shui of their rented house was so bad; I could not rectify it and suggested that they look for another house with better feng shui. I tried my best to help them look for one, but after several tries, I too had to give up because every house they intended to rent had the same bad features.

Those destined to have cancer, I believe will have behaviors that make sure they get the cancers – like bad eating habits or living in houses with bad qi so that health is affected; it is all the workings of the karmic forces.

The next logical question is – what can we do about karma? How can we avoid it or heal the cancer patient?

It is certainly of no use to have a theory and not use it to solve issues. Likewise, having deep thoughts on cancer and the real cause but without a solution is pointless. I will now try to unfold to you how to deal with it.

If you accept the idea of a karmic cause, then there is no use feeling so much anger anymore, you now know that you are just harvesting whatever you had sowed years ago or even in a previous life time. Negative emotions like anger, frustrations, depression, hatred and worries all do nothing good. They embed you in deeper problems such as your immune system being jeopardized, making matters worse, as then, cancer cells can march on unimpeded and relentlessly.

You need not ask God "Why me, of all people!" The answer is clear and it is not necessary to waste time wallowing in that question anymore. You know the reason you contracted this disease and now you can focus your mind, your attention, and energy towards something more useful.

Once you accept your condition, it is so much easier for you to deal with the problem at hand. Firstly, once you acknowledge the diagnosis, sometimes miraculously, you get healed. This is because as far as some souls are concerned, they have learned a lesson and it's now to focus on another lesson plan.

Secondly, you now use your energy to look for ways to get cured rather than fighting the diagnosis, refusing to accept the verdict and forgetting to overcome the disease. If it was bad karma that landed you in such trouble, then the right thing to do is to stop generating more bad vibes! Stop the rot, in other words turn over a new leaf.

This shift in your mental attitude will change your vibration to a higher level causing events and situations to flow smoothly.

I know some will argue, 'What's the point?'

They may feel that because they are currently suffering with cancer and if they perform 'good' acts now, isn't it a bit too late? I believe this type of thinking is wrong and detrimental and keeps people stuck in their decaying thoughts which manifest as a decaying body.

Once you accept responsibility for what you have attracted in this life time, you can change your circumstances now! You don't have to wait until your next life to do so.

If you are not willing to look within and accept your part in contracting the disease this is a selfish attitude towards yourself, where do you think you are heading to? How can your body start healing if you are narrow minded and blame others or the Universe for what you have manifested and attracted on your own. In this case it is best you remain right where you are and cope with the cancer destroying your body all by your self.

Have you ever spoken to someone with cancer? Have you ever noticed how negative some are, how selfish, and how poisonous their minds can be? I have observed this in many cancer cases, and said to myself, 'It is no wonder some of these people have attracted a vicious disease that attacks the body. If one spends their lives attacking and blaming others, being angry with the world and especially self loathing and angry towards self, it doesn't surprise me that they attract a harmful angry disease.

Attitudes must change, people should have a better out look on life and they should stop the blame game and pointing fingers at every one, including God. If any fingers are to be pointed, they should be directed at self. Then one should embrace all shortcomings and change them. People can heal by having a better, more positive way of thinking.

By accepting the condition and coming to terms with it, this allows the healing process to start. When peoples' attitudes change for the better, when even being faced with cancer they can still think about the welfare of others and especially themselves they can set an example to many. When others notice how benevolent a cancer sufferer can be, they may make an effort to examine themselves and change. All good work will not go unnoticed by the Lords of Karma.

With a change in attitude, circumstances may also change. Sufferers who no longer feel like victims may then meet a very good team of health professionals, who will help and work out something for them, like recommending the best and correct drug combinations.

Even if the cancer is not cured, but because the issues have been accepted, changed for the better, it becomes easier to cope with in every situation and the sufferings are lessened. This in itself is a good real time reward.

Take a look at some pictures of cancer eating away at various parts of the body or at some patients in this condition; notice that it is literally rotting away; the foul smell that accompanies cancer patients is unmistakeable.

This is the physical manifestation of some really rotten things that one may have done in lives before. As above, so below – was once said by Hermes Trimegastus. If you are able to see the aura of people, then you will know even better! These people possess some of the darkest auras emanating from their faces and bodies.

I am not able to see auras at will, but sometimes my vibration shifts to a higher gear and my feng shui eyes can see a lot of things! One of my workers had a very black aura emanating from her face. I suddenly noticed this for a brief second only. I was taken aback momentarily. Auras don't lie, that is my firm belief and as she was leading a life of darkness the energy inevitably accompanied her.

So you can see why even with a very healthy lifestyle, good diet, taking health supplements, exercise and medical check ups, one may still get cancer due to past deeds.

Correcting our way of life to one in harmony with the Universe is the best option and one that promises a better life for all both now and in the future.

It is the myopic attitudes of humans that lead to their downfall. We are actually more than our physical self – we have two other components – the Mind and Soul. Mind is the consciousness and soul is the spark from the greater Source, which is eternal. In the real world, there is no time or space. In our world of Maya, or Illusion, we experience linear time, space and distance.

I have accepted the concepts of being an eternal Spirit, and so in my reality, there is no death, only a transformation of beingness. It is just not possible to have only one lifetime to achieve perfection; it is simply not logical come to think of it. I have thus no fear of death. Knowing that what I think, feel and do now will benefit my tomorrow, it makes sense to consciously attract what I want; it's as simple as that.

The Chinese have their own explanation of diseases, including cancers – it is the blockage of energy flow, leading to an imbalance of yin-yang and therefore disharmony, followed by all types of ailments.

A blocked channel means there will be an accumulation of waste and toxic by-products of metabolism and reduced nutrient flow, thus compromising all types of cell function. With deteriorating function, the all important yin-yang balance of health is tipped over to that of a disease causing environment.

Thus, to correct this imbalance, the blockage must be relieved or new channels opened. Surgery, chemotherapy and radiotherapy do nothing to unblock the channels and it is not surprising at all that they are of little or no contribution to the five year survival rates.

Actually, with the severance of channels using these procedures, the patient is often further compromised. Whether or not this theory is correct, there is so far no herbal concoction that has a significant advantage over these treatments either. This again brings us back to square one. Or does it?

As mentioned earlier, I had to look into the spiritual aspect to get a hint of the answer, since Western and Eastern medical science is of not much help. The answer must be able to explain all known facts and data of cancer occurrence and behavior. I have a theory; it may not lead to a direct cure but I feel it is far better than that for it leads to being able to keep anything too harmful at bay and possible prevention of disease ever seriously occurring.

My proposal is as follows. It is for all of us, whether we have cancer or not. We keep the body – which some refer to as our temple as clean as possible, in thought, word and deed from now on. We provide ourselves with wholesome nutrition mainly from the vegetable kingdom and the fish kingdom.

The health of the gut must be taken care of i.e.: by daily bowel movements, we must do our best to avoid constipation at all costs, and to achieve this we should take some foods or supplements with the right kinds of friendly bacteria. This will be discussed in more detail in another chapter.

It is really important to steer away from negative emotions such as sorrow, hatred, jealousy, anger and ideas of revenge and instead imbibe good positive thoughts and emotion. You may want to do some form of social work or charity contributions to improve your spiritual wealth. Then let the Tao flow as it is, face whatever Life throws at you and accept it gladly. Meditate and meditate!

See yourself as a healthy person. Imagine the physical problems slowly being dissolved away in your mind's eye. Follow the doctor's advice to the extent that you are able. Know that really you are an eternal Being. May the Blessings be!!

A Brief Summary...

Let me be more specific, as some readers may still be confused as to what are my real suggestions, since this is an important chapter. To put it in a simple way, the following paragraph should summarize my concepts thus far:–

Those diagnosed with any cancer at Stage 1 stand the best chance with medical treatment by their oncologists mainly because treatment at this stage is still not that invasive and destructive.

Those with Stage 2 cancers, well, to me are at the watershed area, since they still can opt for the medical approach.

Those with Stage 3 onwards, I think medical treatment may not really work that much in their favor and also the cost of the medication tends to escalate at this stage. One would need a very strong belief in themselves, the medication and total trust in the Universe in order to have successful results. I am not saying it is impossible, it most certainly can be.

I know of so many cases and stories of families, especially the poor and middle class who have spent their hard earned savings trying various medical treatments or on quacks and charlatans and yet their loved one still succumbs to the cancer within months.

It is tough on a family who have decided to spend that much money to find that at the end they are left with barely any funds on top of the grief of losing a loved one. It sounds harsh but sometimes I feel for the surviving members of the families who have spent all their savings on medication and are left with bills that it would be better to save the money for education and use by the surviving family members. I say this because I see the bigger picture and know that if their family members have not used any type of emotional healing or belief work on top of the physical healing there is not much chance that they will survive.

Energy and Healing...

If people want to overcome this disease I would say the best option is to go the holistic way. This is also recommended for those receiving medical treatments and for those serious in improving their health and immunity. I would suggest eating more fruits and vegetables, less meat and processed foods, also to do a detoxification program for their bowels, liver, kidneys and blood systems.

The hardest part is to change their mindset and thinking – they would need to detox the brain as well as physically detoxing the body and to improve upon their nutrition seriously with supplements and nourishing meals.

The wholesome nutrition mentioned in the above paragraph will be expanded in the chapters on Supplements. In fact, with each of the suggestions given, a few chapters will be needed to describe the rationale behind them which can be found further on in this book.

Energy is the very basic requirement of all living organisms. When our energy levels are down, so too is our immune system, this makes us vulnerable to attacks from bacteria and viruses. The Hindu yogis and Chinese metaphysicians knew much about energy, which they called prana or qi respectively.

The chakra system and the system of acupuncture meridians describe the energy map of the body precisely. It would be a monumental task to explain both systems in detail but I just wanted to bring these two issues up for you readers to know about their existence and how they actually compliment each other.

In the study of Anatomy, these two systems are non–existent as there are no equivalent anatomical structures, microscopic or macroscopic. This is the issue I want to emphasise – those who only use their physical eyes as senses, will only discover as far as the eyes can see. The yogi and the Taoist masters, however, use their intuition, meditation and their "third eye" to investigate and they can see much more!

Acupuncture points and energy meridians must be true because western doctors still use acupuncture in very extensive clinical settings, especially as an anaesthetic, and yet the meridians are invisible to the eyes.

Chakra energy healing has been practiced by many Energy Healers but the scientific community continues to ignore their contributions.

Thus if we are to defeat cancer, we must understand energy mechanics very well. If we are to improve our immune system, again we have to harness energy. Energy can be positive or negative, so be careful of which energy you absorb. To make life easier for readers - a brief description of the systems is given in chapters that follow.

There is another fact that indirectly proves the existence of the acupuncture meridians and this comes from an unlikely source. Some shamans of South America were asked to draw, on the body, of what they perceived were the energy lines they knew of. One of the shaman's then obliged and with a marker pen, drew the energy lines on a person's body. A photograph was taken and later compared with the Chinese acupuncture meridians. This was shown to be almost an exact replica of the Chinese acupuncture charts.

Now the shamans were so called illiterate medicine men in South America and they had never heard of acupuncture and meridians, yet what they could see was almost exactly the same as established acupuncture points and meridian lines.

Of course this sort of proof is unscientific, scientists are not able to plot the energy lines and do not even think they exist. So if we are to keep waiting for scientific proof and statistical evidence, I think we would be left far behind in the expansion of our thinking and personal growth not to mention the world's evolution.

Before going into the chakra and other energy based topics, I wish to spend some time explaining what is actually meant by energy as I think to understand energy is to know the essence behind everything!

Since I have had training in Chinese metaphysics, my ideas of energies have also expanded. I do see a lot of things very differently from many people and as I have already mentioned, especially since I opened my feng shui eyes.

The Chinese use mainly two types of calendars – one is lunar based and the other, solar based. The major populace use the lunar while very few use the solar, otherwise known as the Hsia calendar unless they have been trained to use it.

Now let me show you why nowadays I use the Hsia calendar, and so where everyone is crazy celebrating the New Year i.e.: 1st January, I am not too bothered about it as it has not much meaning in terms of energy.

Everyone should remember the tsunami that hit many parts of the world in 2004. It was so destructive and devastating, bringing death to many on its path. I had just passed by the beach front in Batu Ferringhi, on the island of Penang, less than an hour before the huge wave struck, killing many picnickers.

I had no idea as I was still driving on my way to do a feng shui audit for a client. I was caught in a terrible jam along a road that should not have been so grid locked at that time. I was puzzled until I received a phone call from my sister in Sydney. She had seen news footage of a devastating tsunami and was warned it could hit Penang Island after the destruction it had caused in India, Sri Lanka and The Maldives.

It was 26th December, 2004. In terms of the Chinese way of thinking, the date can be translated as – Yang Earth/ Tiger (Yang Wood) day, in the year of Yang Wood Monkey(Yang Metal) with Flying Star Number 5 in the Central Palace.

Of course this would make absolutely no sense to many people but to those who know feng shui and to me it says a lot about the energy present at that point in time. For a start, the year has the 'bad' number 5 in Chinese metaphysics. It signifies earth disasters, calamities and so on.

So this indicated to me a disaster having something to do with the earth element, for example it may involve a volcano or an earthquake. An earthquake under the sea will result in a tsunami no doubt. So that part of the prediction was true. The year was that of a Wood energy, and wood destroys earth in Chinese metaphysics, so the clash of wood with earth had been set up. The wood in that year, Yang Wood, is big wood, so the wood is a match for the powerful earth.

That day was a day of Earth Tiger. Tigers clash with Monkeys under the Chinese zodiac signs, so another conflict had been set up – day clashing with year. With two sets of clashes, the perfect disaster scene had been set.

The energy for 27th December was described in the Chinese Almanac, as the energy of death. No wonder, when we woke up the next morning, the papers had headlines of death. The Chinese Hsia calendar has a lot of meanings and values which can be interpreted by those who know how to understand and apply this knowledge while the calendar the world uses, only tells the year, month and day.

Once you understand energy, its laws and application, you will be able to understand the Universe. To the Chinese scholars, time is cyclical, in small and large cycles of 12, 60 and 180 year cycles. However to most, with the calendar that everyone is so familiar, time seems to be linear.

Linear time is really an illusion; I say this because it is so one dimensional while we are currently living in a 3D world! Let us look at other years where the number 5 is in the central palace in feng shui calculations. The most infamous one was that of 1941, Year of the Metal Snake. This was the beginning of the 2nd World War. The war ended in 1945, Year of the Wood Rooster, with number 1 as the Flying star number, this number signifies water, which is calm.

The 1st World War, in 1914 also had the number 5 earth and it was the Year of the Wood Tiger. Here, the wood of the year and the wood of the tiger combined to clash with the number 5 earth, oh, what a big clash it was. The wood in both cases was Yang – two ferocious males, and so the Yin-Yang balance was destroyed, there could not be any harmony. The world had to go to war.

The next number 5 year will be 2013, Year of Water Snake. I hope it will be a non-event number 5 as in years gone by with no worldly problems. However, some rumors suggest that it may not be that peaceful.

These rumors were started by the Mayans, who had a calendar system that was started on 13th August 3113 BC and ends on 21st December 2012. There are two schools of thought here one of which is that to the Mayans, it was useless to continue their calendar because they had predicted a major catastrophe.

Their time calculation is also based on a cyclical concept and their one cycle is 5,125.4 years. Their end date coincides with their 13th baktun cycle. Notice the number 13. To the Mayans, the crucial year will be 2012 but for Chinese metaphysicians, it is more likely that

2013, the year with the unlucky number 5 star and Year of Water Snake is the year to be careful about.

The other school of thought is the group who believe the Mayan calendar ends on the same date but it won't be a cataclysmic ending. As we have read the Mayan's believed in circular time, with every end signifying a new beginning. Their belief is that the Mayans felt 2012 will be a time of purification, a fresh start where we will all reconnect with the energy of love. It is said to be the beginning of a new and unwritten cycle but this time from a higher plane of existence where contrasts will be smaller and manifestation quicker.

Those who believe in catastrophe may end up in a tsunami, earth quake or volcano and those who believe in the energy of love will always be in the right place at the right time.

We all have a choice about what to believe in 2012, large numbers will believe none of it, others will be filled with doom and gloom, preaching 'The end of the world is nigh' while many will see the coming of The Age Of Aquarius, a whole new world and a new dimension of wisdom, divine love, peace and understanding.

This book is not about the year 2012 or its predictions. I just wanted to show that energy physics is so important in order to understand everything. If energy is the universe, then our body, also thriving on energy, must follow some basic principle or plan, and medicine today has not accepted energy as the yogi, shaman, Taoist or Buddhists have done.

The energies that modern medicine understands are the likes of calories, the biochemical Krebs cycle and electron transfer chain, chemicals like phosphates and oxidation – reduction potentials. How much has this knowledge contributed to the over all understanding of human physiology?

According to the scientists and much of the world, it has contributed a great deal and they are awarded the Noble Prize for their discoveries.

According to me, nothing much while great eastern masters who have discovered greater truths are left unknown and unappreciated.

Going back to what I was talking of earlier about the energy behind dates and times, here is a more recent example, since many people have such short memories! There was an act of terrorism in Pakistan on 3rd March 2009 where some dozen or so men ambushed and killed six police escorts of the visiting Sri Lankan cricket team and the brave bus driver. They had used rifles, grenades and rocket launches in the attack. The cricketers were lucky to have escaped death but seven players, an umpire and a coach were wounded in the attack. It shocked every one.

On that day, the energy was very bad as it is known as the year breaker energy. In every Chinese almanac they have calculated where the year breakers are – this means the energy of the year verses the energy of the universe – in other words a very powerful clash. What happened in Sri Lanka was of course world news. In Malaysia, we also experienced some upheaval in the energy on that day; some unusual but minor disputes were recorded and deemed newsworthy locally.

The malevolent energy of the day had also acted in the local scene in the town where I stay. There was a bad motor vehicular accident on the road near my place and the accident victim's blood was spilled over the road. This example of traumatic occurrences on the same day at world, national and local levels validates what I believe; that the Chinese calendar has more information than many will know.

The above discussions on the measurement of time by the various cultures have touched on several aspects. However I wish to relate my own special experience of time in an incident when I believe time was slowed down. It was back in the years when I was studying at our local university as an under graduate. I was on my motorbike and was rushing back to the hostel for lunch. I took a short cut through the campus and negotiated a sharp bend when suddenly I saw a car right in front of me.

I had no time to react to avoid a sure accident. However something strange happened. I saw everything in slow motion – I saw myself being hit by the car and flying into the air straight towards the windscreen of the oncoming car. I could see the driver holding both arms up to protect himself. Then, as suddenly as this vision had come, it disappeared and I found myself still on my bike. It was then that I sensed I could avoid the deadly accident and tried my luck. At the last moment, I managed to swerve my bike to the left, at the same time the driver also realized it was possible to evade impact and he swerved in the opposite direction. We missed each other by seconds and inches. I am sure that many others have reported or experienced the slowing of time.

Now that we know energy is all that is to life, let me discuss other forms of energy regarded as healing. This is more closely related to the subject of cancers than about wars and natural disasters.

I believe there are basically two types of healing energy – one directly from the Universe and the other being that generated by the healers themselves.

Let me discuss the first type. There are several such as Universal healing energy, Reiki etc. Basically the practitioners act as channels for the healing energy to be discharged through them.

I am a Reiki practitioner myself. However I use it very sparingly for many reasons which I will share now. First allow me to describe how others use this tool and their understanding of it. There are now many such people who are doing Reiki either voluntarily or as an occupation.

When I got into Reiki, it was hardly heard of by people in my country. I have friends and I have seen many others who went into a healing spree in many such healing camps organized by numerous organizations. Lots of healers are truly doing it to help the sick but they are unaware of the many repercussions.

I believe there are hazards involved when working with energy. The worst is to absorb the negative energies of the receiver. Many are not told of this in energy work. It is important that all students of energy healing be taught to ground and protect themselves first and then to cleanse themselves afterwards. This is very basic in all energy work and once done Reiki can be applied and used without harmful effects.

Then, an indirect effect is to lead people to believe that they will be cured and thus they neglect proper medical attention. All energy healers should be told never to diagnose and if they suspect something amiss to recommend that their client goes to the doctor. Also we must never ask someone to stop taking a prescribed medication.

The founder of Reiki had made another discovery that in trying to help the masses, he actually led them astray – they were really cured of their illness but instead of going to work for a living, these people continued to beg for alms. He had thought that after healing them of their illnesses for free, they would go back to their families or start to work and earn an honest living. He was disillusioned. He then made a rule that practitioners are to perform the healing only when it is requested of them and there should be a payment of money or an energy exchange. He believed that when one is charged for the service, receivers of such healing would not take it for granted.

The second category of energy healer I mentioned belongs to Qigong masters for example, who use their own qi to heal others. It is very tiring work indeed and if they are not careful, they too may absorb the negative energies of their clients. If they do not charge themselves up by meditating and doing their own special exercises for this purpose, their immune systems may be compromised and thus they too might expose themselves to pathogens.

Anyway, as I believe that cancers are mostly karmic in nature, correct me if I am wrong but no amount of Reiki or Universal energies can heal them. That is another reason why I don't practise such healings unless in special circumstances. Once I had a good friend - a lady doctor, she was dying of lung cancer although she was not a smoker. She was in severe pain. I practised Reiki on her to alleviate some distress and pain and it certainly worked, but only for shorter and shorter periods.

The experience was very deep, she described how she felt someone using an instrument to bore holes into her liver (where there were the metastases) after which she felt relieved and more at peace. I know that the angel guides were at work, although she never saw these guides or spirit healers.

As I was working in another town, I could only give her some relief for a few days and when I returned, she passed away not long after that. Thus even energy healing does not help cure cancers.

My other experience was when I did healing for another friend who was very psychic. She did not have any ailments but was willing to receive the energy. Although her eyes were closed, she gave me a running commentary of how she felt and of what she saw. One of the visions she had was a woman spirit guide and at another time she saw a man who looked like an Indian chief with a full head dress of feathers. Each session involved different spirit guides.

I do believe however that Reiki can have an indirect effect on healing a cancer sufferer. By helping to alleviate pain, make one relaxed, at peace and feel happier this can help a person let go more easily or find the will to live.

Most of you may have heard of Sai Baba of India. Many think of him as a fake and con artist but I have a very different experiences that tells me otherwise. I have a cousin who is very close to Sai Baba and she would organize trips to India for many cancer patients to undergo healing.

She said some were healed while others were not and some even died while in India. She had very trying times when this occurred because to make arrangements to bring the bodies back to Malaysia involves a lot of red tape. To prevent false hope and such wasted trips, for most of these trips are funded by the patients themselves, she had devised a plan agreeable to Sai.

She would send to him the names of each patient and Sai would only recommend those who were destined to benefit from the trip, thus saving untold miseries. The point I want to make is this, even the Sai himself is unable to save many cancer stricken patients, although there were cases when he said "Your cancer is cancelled" and it was.

He must have known that some of these must bear their own karma for their own good. Sometimes, the Sai Baba himself is taken ill from all the healings he performs. Few know the reason which is he has to take on their karma to heal them, so he has really suffered a lot. The karmic energy has to be manifested. Now in the light of what I have discussed, what can medicine do?

I do not want to bring no hope to cancer patients, it seems so pessimistic. Rather the message to be conveyed is that one has to do something, be it medicinal or prayer, in the hope that it helps to alleviate some sufferings. Perhaps, by the grace of God, the patient may even be healed, as the saying goes; God helps those who help themselves.

I have mentioned prayers above and would ask you to be open minded as I dwell further on this significant topic. I believe prayers are important but many don't realise how to make them effective! Most people turn to prayer from a place of sadness, desperation and despair with prayer as their only hope. They pray for their loved ones like "Dear God, please make him well again." In this type of prayer, there are several nuances. As heartless as it sounds, in the above prayer the person really is praying only for their own good because they don't want to lose their loved one and are afraid he or she will leave them forever.

There is nothing wrong with praying for ones own good but we cannot take away another's free will. Also I believe it is important to find the essence behind the prayer. If one prays for material gain based on the essence of greed, lack or fear this is not a 'real' prayer. Prayers of love for everybody's gain or benefit are prayers that may be answered. The crucial ingredients in any prayer are that we must feel deeply; we can use our imagination to visualise and we must have the belief and trust that our visions will be made manifest. However the ultimate secret key to prayer is that if we are not happy we will never get what we want.

I would ask you to stop for a moment to reflect if what I say is the basic truth. Next, many do not know the truth behind the cancers. If the ingredients of prayer mentioned above are followed and the request is uttered in such a way as "Dear God, I leave it to you to decide what is best for our loved one. Let Thy Will be done"

This to me is better because first we acknowledge that in matters of life and death, the Higher Authority has a lot of clout. Second, we recognize that the person having the cancer has his own plans, usually well mapped out even before birth. We thus do not impose our own will on anyone.

Here we have followed the principles of the Tao. As earlier mentioned it is important to be happy and feel deeply in you that God has heard your sincere prayer and will respond. Then leave it as what will be, will be. You may not always get exactly what you have asked for but you will definitely receive something and some times it is essentially more than you could even think possible.

To my thinking, God has given us the most precious gift – that of our own free will. We can do whatever we like; the consequences that follow are another matter. But if we surrender our will to Him, it is another great gift from us.

I had mentioned about emotions being an important component in the cause of cancers and ill health. Western medicine has neglected this aspect, especially in the case of cancers. Thus all the oncologists will attack this by their ever expanding array of very specific anti-cancer drugs of increasing potencies and not look into the root cause like the link with some emotional behaviors and address them.

However, Dr Edward Bach ventured where no medical doctor has been before – by believing that health depends on being in harmony with our souls. The strategy was to address the negative emotions like depression, anxiety and emotional traumas that are thought to obstruct the body's own healing abilities. Dr Bach spent an entire life time researching natural antidotes and he came up with his Bach Flower Remedies. It is indeed interesting to see that he was brave enough to go against main stream medicine to suggest that people with cancers have the following personalities or emotional behaviors, with the remedies in brackets –

(a) Blaming others especially own kids – cancer of reproductive organs [chicory]
(b) Hatred, jealousy, envy and depressed – most cancers [holly]
(c) Always blaming oneself, no self love – female cancers [pine]
(d) Power – hungry tyrants; guards, police and immigration types [vine]
(e) Always breaks promises, domineering parents – lung cancer [walnut]

The beautiful part of using Bach Flower Therapy is that it has no side effects at all, it works at the level of subtle energies, has no need to adhere to strict dosages , it is non-addictive, gentle in action and age is no bar. It does not interact with any medication and thus can be used in conjunction with anti-cancer drugs.

I use Bach Flower therapy whenever a case demands it and if the patient is open to such ideas. I have a set of the Bach flower remedies and when I first ran my hand over the little bottles, scanning for energy,

I was really surprised. I could feel numerous tingling sensations over my hand; in fact it was like the feeling of energy pulses hitting my palm.

Not only did I have this experience but I also got a mental impression of many of these flower essences screaming at me for attention!! Like little children all talking to me at once. Before embarking on my spiritual journey I was not aware of such sensations but now it could mean that my senses are getting more sensitive to energy of late.

Although a lot of praise should go to Dr Bach, many Asian cultures also have the same concept. We are so familiar with the term - "Go have a Seven Flower Bath" when we are facing some very trying times.

Thus, it is of small wonder why some people who have a good sense of humor, and laugh a lot, live longer. In some parts of the world, they have Laughing Clubs where members would meet and just laugh and laugh. As for me, whenever I have a chance to laugh at a joke or funny incident, I make sure I laugh heartily.

The Bach Flower therapy is a link to Nature's secrets. It gives me a hint that Nature has a cure for every disease on earth but some are yet to be discovered, or accepted by the medical community; and yet some are deliberately suppressed because the people involved are unable to make money out of them.

Perhaps an example is the Graviola tree of South America. The natives of the land have been using it for hundreds of years to cure their ailments. After spending so much on its research and being unable to synthesize the potent factor under laboratory conditions, the company gave up as it could not be patented.

How can you patent the fruit of any tree that grows so abundantly and freely in nature and is available to all? In my mind, nature is willing to give up its deepest secrets but due to human's selfishness and greed for money, the secrets have been held back until humans evolve to a higher level – one that thinks of universal values. It shows that we must not be selfish and keep what good we have discovered to ourselves but to share with others. Until then, many need to suffer in order to work out their karma.

There is another form of cancer then – the cancer of human society that is sick. Each cell represents a human being and just as each man is for himself, each cancer cell is also for itself without sharing the nutrients of the body, in the concept of survival of the fittest.

The lies, back stabbing, hatred, jealousy, greed and racist attitudes result in a society that is divided and in disarray, finally law and order crumbles. The environment is polluted with both physical garbage and bad qi and finally the world too becomes eroded, just like cancer cells killing the host. The cancer of corruption is another form of cancer in society. Corruption will destroy everything in its path – both the corrupt officials as well as those who bribe.

So, do we need more weapons of mass destruction to stop this rot, do we require stronger, more specific and toxic chemotherapeutic agents? The answer is no, what the world needs is Love for all mankind and life on this planet. Don't you see the parallel here – the microcosm and macrocosm? The approach our politicians and scientists use is all wrong, both in the micro and macrocosms. Small wonder they have not solved the basic issues.

Though I have given my views on cancer there is another aspect I wish to introduce. This is a real surprise to me as well. It is really something new to me even, although it is in parallel to my line of thinking. This was reported by Brandon Bays. She uses a unique style to release pent up energies of people to heal them of their physical illness.

One gentleman by the name of Jim was referred to her because he wanted to know why he had lung cancer. Jim was given three months to live by his doctor but he has survived way beyond that. He however took every treatment the doctors suggested both chemotherapy and radiotherapy. His tumor had not regressed as it was expected to and the latest MRI showed only a smaller shadow in the affected lung. It was at this stage when he sought Brandon Bays' help to find out why he had this cancer.

It was during the therapy that the cause for the aggressive lung cancer came to light .A memory flashed through Jim. He was taken care of by his young mother after his father left them. It was while in school that bombs were dropped in wartime Europe and sensing something, he broke free from his school teachers and ran to look for his mother. He could not find her but after some searching, he eventually found his mother and kept shaking her body to wake her up. Finally a policeman came and told him that his mother was dead and pulled him away.

Young Jim was only sixteen then. He felt great rage at God and against the enemies for taking his mother's life away. How could this have happened? He was then asked by the therapist to forgive all that he had been so angry with over his mother's death. He was told that no one could be taken away before their time and that the enemy soldiers were just obeying orders from their superiors.

He duly let go all the hatred and rage that had been in his body for over 50 years. Thus he knew the reason for his cancer, and he let the bad energies of hatred go, he forgave all.

After the session with the therapist, Jim had an appointment with the doctors and another scan was done, this time there was no trace of the cancerous growth in the lungs at all. His doctors accredited it to the new chemotherapy regime that was given to Jim two years ago while other doctors thought that the original diagnosis must have been a mistake. This typical reaction by the medical community is understandable – for their level of awareness.

As this case was so unique with documentary proof of biopsies and scans and being followed up by reputable doctors, it was recorded in a medical journal. But for a Jim, he knew the reason why. In fact he was reported to be more happy and docile, no more getting angry and upset at the most trivial of things.

Forgiveness is one of the greatest medicines of all times. It is free, no side effects and always available. Just by forgiving the person who has hurt you, is a huge step on the road to recovery. Love and forgiveness is the secret to a happy and healthy life. Simply by applying these two secret weapons, wars will end. They will end the very moment we all forgive one another and start building up society, rather than destroying each other. Love really conquers all. It is possible – if every one decides not to go to war, who will fight with who?

Cancer Diets are unfortunately also useless. There are several groups, professionals and health experts who have devised their own diet theories for cancer patients to follow with a few claims of success. However the latest report from World Cancer Research Fund has cautioned cancer patients to be aware that unfortunately none will help to prolong lives or help cure cancers as claimed.

Diets that advocate vegetarian or vegan regimes that are said to rid the body of toxins and so lead to a cure are actually dangerous. If patients carry out the food regimes strictly they will have a very imbalanced diet which actually makes matters worse. The Gerson therapy which claims to cleanse the body and boost metabolism is particularly dubious as a number of patients suffered nausea, perforated colon and infections from the enemas.

I heard some of my readers asking if cancer will ever be cured at all. From what I have written, I may make it seem very bleak indeed. In my vision, I see that cancers can be conquered to a large extent by advancements in science but not mainly medical science. If scientists keep on devising new types of chemotherapeutic agents, then there will not be very significant advances.

Some answers lie in energy medicine, which will then be electromagnetic in nature. However, in all treatment modalities, the cancer patients rely on some other's work or discovery. This is only part of the story. He or she must do something themselves. They should change their rigid mind sets, bad attitudes and habits, radiate love and compassion and do meritorious deeds and yet not claim for recognition.

The body can heal itself; you can heal yourself, but your efforts are required, be it meditation, special prayers or by asking for Divine help. You will have to be involved in your own healing journey. Heed the message of Lord Buddha, who attained Enlightenment by his own efforts.

9. Dealing with Death

As doctors wanting to heal the sick we have to face the fact that we will encounter those heart breaking times when no matter what we do for someone, they still die. This topic is very important as it was never very well treated while I was in medical school. We were given the impression that we could save all our patients, when in the real world as a houseman I saw so many die right in front of my eyes; I felt quite disillusioned at times. I remember two cases very well.

I was still a medical student but was assigned to ward duty. One case I had was a poor farmer in very bad shape; he was old, skinny and frail. The next case was a young, tall and well built man from a rich family. After a few days I was shocked to learn that the young man had died while the old farmer had survived and was discharged back to his village. I could still remember their faces. This experience shook me to the very core. They both had perforated appendicitis; the young man was admitted first as he was a city dweller while the old farmer took several days to be admitted and his operation was even further delayed. In both surgeries I was assisting the surgeon and both operations went well. The results were a complete shock to both me and the surgeon.

I also know of many doctors who think they are so smart and tell their patients something like "I'm afraid your cancer is advanced and I believe you have only six months to live." However these doctors are often incorrect and what a surprise they get when they see their terminal patients at the airport terminal going for vacation number three a few years after their terminal predictions!

We want our patients to put their trust and faith in us but it is comments like these that cause the most harm to those that do. They believe the doctor completely and it can become a self fulfilling prophecy. The rebels who like a challenge are the ones that say – 'No way! I'm going to prove my doctor wrong!' They are the ones who end up surviving! Is this really what we want as doctors? I don't think so!

I have learned never to be that smart as far as foretelling what will happen to my so called terminal cases. The least I can do is to give them some hope, but never false hope. I let them know there is a glimmer of hope should they undergo modern cancer treatments rather than untested products that have only testimonies but no scientific backing.

To many people, a diagnosis of cancer means lots of suffering, pain both physical and emotional and death. To have a broader outlook, death can strike at anytime; the very young can die, so too can the healthy from accidents and natural disasters and so on.

Although as a doctor we have many patients who die under our care, we have very little interaction with the families other than to inform them of the bad news. In one case, I had the rare opportunity to interact with the family as I was a close family friend. The experience I gained was really an eye opener. My association with this family was from my school days and although I had left many years earlier, I kept in touch with the Principal and his family.

One day I received an email from the daughter that her father was dying and had wanted to see me urgently. He requested this when they transferred him back from Singapore to live his last days in the town he loved so much.

When I went to see him, the daughter took me aside and pleaded with me to help her father recover. Actually there was nothing anyone could do. I said I would see what information I could get from my psychic friend in South Africa. I contacted this lady and she told me she saw that the silver cord of the patient had been cut and thus it was time for him to go. So really there was nothing we could do. The strategy was to prepare the family for the inevitable. When I told them the news, although so disappointed, they now changed their thinking into making him as comfortable as possible.

However I was still not satisfied and even in my dreams, I asked God for an answer. In one particular dream, I was tiny when compared to two very large giant footprints, which represented God and as I looked up, I could see only the sky and nothing. I knew God had answered me by giving me a message in my mind – 'Don't worry about him, he has to continue his journey, let him go'. I really felt so much better once I had a direct answer from God Almighty.

I did my best to prepare the family but to my surprise, my ex-principle had done the job himself. He was lucid one moment and unconscious the next and he drifted in and out like that for at least a week. This was partly due to the morphine but I believed this was not the case because the family had requested minimal sedation and I needed to use Reiki at times to soothe him.

When he was conscious, he would tell of a journey that he was undertaking, how he crossed some rivers in a boat, and how far he had yet to travel in this very wonderful land. He was meeting some of his long gone relatives and friends on his journey; he knew it was his last. This narrative by him gave me several insights into life after death for I believed his on off unconsciousness was when his soul travelled in the after world. Not long after I left him to go back to work, I got a phone call to say he passed away in his sleep.

I have another experience that I wish to relate. I heard that my auntie was not feeling so well and I made a trip to pay her a visit. As soon as I took one look at her, I asked my relatives to get her admitted as she was in quite a bad condition with a high fever and urinary tract infection. She was over 80 years old and bed ridden.

When the doctors examined her, they immediately put her into intensive care. At this time, I was a very much more experienced feng shui practitioner and had increased my knowledge of feng shui tremendously. I noticed the bed number she was assigned to but more than that, I saw so many shar qi (poison arrows) pointing at her. For an old lady, so frail in health and in severe infection, this would be a huge stumbling block in her recovery.

I tried to get her to another bed, with a more favorable number and no shar qi (negative energy) pointing at her. She was duly moved and I felt very optimistic for her and so happy to be able to use my extra knowledge. The next day I heard they had to shift her back to the original bed because all the intensive monitoring equipment in the new bed had fused. This was really very disturbing to me. I actually had shivers down my spine, as I could feel the message given to me.

Such coincidences do not occur. I knew that her time was up and also that I must not intervene with her fate anymore. I looked at it as a warning to me not to meddle. All I could do was give moral support to the family. In one of my visits, she became stable and just when I left for the trip back to my town, my cousins phoned me to say that my auntie had passed away soon after I left her room.

This was another significant sign to me. In cases where we are very attached to our loved ones, they will only leave us when we are not around as it makes their leaving less traumatic. Have you ever heard stories like this before? My aunt always looked up to me because I cared for her and gave her and her family so much medical advice and medication. Although it was her time she may have felt it would be more difficult to leave while I was still in the room.

In traumatic and sudden death, it is very different. I would like to give my comments here. In these situations, the suddenness of the death can cause resentment in the person's soul as his life is snatched away from him. In many cases, they do not even know that they have died. This was very much seen in the aftermath of the tsunami of 2004. My friend whose family knew of a taxi driver friend reported that he had picked up two Europeans in town who had asked to be taken to the airport. However upon reaching the airport, the two passengers had disappeared from the backseat of his taxi.

In Phuket, Thailand, this same story is heard and even more stories of hearing people crying around the beach but no one can be seen. The same was in Aceh, Indonesia as we have friends who had gone there as volunteers to help rehabilitate the survivors. They reported seeing a woman running around asking people to help her baby and she would just disappear suddenly. If their souls do not rest in peace, this nightmare keeps recurring. They will be trapped in time and be neither here nor there.

I wish to relate another story told to me by my Feng Shui Grandmaster. He had gone to USA on an assignment and was driven from the airport to the residence of the man who had hired him. On the way, they drove through the countryside and the driver stopped a while for some snacks. Then Grandmaster encountered a group of Native American Indians asking for his help to send them to their happy hunting ground.

Grandmaster was not taken by surprise because he sees and communicates with lost souls. He was unprepared however, so he told them he would come back this way in a few days time and do the needful. All the while, the driver who was sent to pick him up thought it was funny this old Chinese man talking to himself.

On his way back to the airport, he told the driver to stop at the same spot and he took out his Taoist paraphernalia of joss sticks, candles and prayer papers he got from Chinatown and started to pray. He saw the same braves with their chief appearing and then a pathway became visible as each of the braves who died in some war against the United States Calvary walked away, thanking Grandmaster one by one as they disappeared. They had all died in battle with no ceremony conducted. Their anguished souls were trapped in time and space and released only when prayers were conducted by Grandmaster.

At the time of my writing, it came to my knowledge that at the 100th anniversary of the death of the legendary Apache warrior Geronimo, his 20 descendants filed a suit asking for his remains to be freed, and along with it, his Spirit. Geronimo died in 1909. His great-grandson, Harlyn Geronimo wanted the remains of Geronimo and the funeral objects to be freed from Fort Still and the other places they were kept (by the Order of Skull and Bones) around 1918. They wanted a true Apache burial as otherwise it is their belief that the spirit is wandering as a lost soul until a proper burial has been performed.

I was actually so saddened to hear of this because I know what his great-grandson said is so true, as exemplified by the story told to me by my Grandmaster. I really hope that after 100 years of suffering, the great spirit of Geronimo will be given due respect as a great warrior and chief and be given the proper burial ceremonies denied thus far. For Geronimo, Ohm mani padme Ohm!!!

I really have very strong beliefs about freeing the spirit of the departed, let me relate another event in USA. There was an air disaster where the entire crew and passengers died. After the wreckage was salvaged and investigated as to the cause of the fatal air crash, the airline company concerned used some of the wrecked airplane's spare parts and fitted them into other aircraft from the same airline.

This re-cycling of usable parts is brilliant but for one fact - no one thought about the dead spirits being attached to the crashed air plane's pieces and hauntings became common in all the planes fitted with the salvaged remains. Crew members sighted glimpses of the dead pilot and co- pilot in their aircraft. From then on, such a policy of re-cycling parts of air crash disasters was banned.

Thus, I do not think it is a good idea that the US builds the Navy assault ship called USS New York, costing about US $1 billion that contains about 7.5 tons of steel from the fallen World Trade Centre. I guess some people have no idea.

All these reports show that we are basically energy and energy can not be destroyed. It just changes from one form to another. So we are souls that inhabit a physical body to experience life on this very dense physical plane. Thus, in reality, there is no death. What is death here is birth into the spiritual world and vice versa.

My psychic friend from South Africa once commented to me that perhaps the Chinese were quite right in one aspect, about giving offerings to their dead relatives who indeed receive them in the astral world! In my own theory, this is why there are many more haunted places in Western society, because of souls being trapped, than in the East as we have several types of ceremonies to send them off! Even with gifts and paper money to spend.

The real point I wish to make here, apart from wandering away from this important message, is that we must let go of our loved ones when they pass over to the other side or we will impede their journey of evolution. One way to let them go is not to display a big photo of them.

It may seem a strange comment but let me relate this story. I was working in London and had a good friend. She told me that ever since her mother had died, she had always felt her presence in the house or a glimpse of her which made her a little nervous. I then noticed a large photo of her mother and I suggested that she put the photo away. This is because such large photos attract the soul to them or a remnant of an energy imprint is captured within the photograph.

My friend took my advice and very soon afterwards she realised that she no longer felt depressed and the house became a lot brighter with no more sightings of her mother.

Can we contact the ones who have departed? This I am sure most will say is possible because contact via a medium has been demonstrated in several cultures across the globe. I feel it is important to state that whatever mediumship people use the mediums attract beings due to their beliefs and communicate through their filters. One must be careful of anything brought through another person. Someone of a low vibration can attract any unknown entity to them and entities from lower planes like to play tricks on us! Once the being has been contacted, firstly the message may not be accurate. Secondly, the being may not be who you think! There is also a high possibility that the medium is not able to contact the loved one and the person seeking this connection may be very sad.

I have been taught that higher communication is not to be encouraged, unless you are at a high and positive vibration to attract a loving energy. I must also warn that playing with Ouija boards is certainly not to be done at all costs. This is because it is a portal where negative entities can gain entry into our world and dimension with untold dangers to all involved. Apart from lost souls, entities of non-human origin and far more dangerous, may be let in.

I think that all contact with the non physical should be from within yourself in that loving place where you are connected to the highest part of you and can therefore attract the same to you.

Sometimes the departed will try to contact their loved ones by way of dreams, giving certain messages blended within the dream. As for me I have dreams of my father at least once every year. There were two occasions of contact which I wish to relate. The most memorable one was when I had qualified as a doctor and was finally going home. My father had passed on while I was a second year medical student and I was only told about it one month after he died, this meant I was not able to attend his send off. I decided to take a slow journey home by ship and on the first night at sea, I had a dream of him. I saw he was looking down at me, with half a smile, proud and happy that I had qualified as a doctor, just like my elder brother.

I woke up from the dream, it was so real. I went to the window and looked out into the night sky and sea. The moon was bright and I could see the waves shimmering under the moon light. I felt it then in my heart that my dad really knew I was finally coming home as a doctor.

The next experience was even more unbelievable. I was then working as a houseman in the district hospital. One afternoon I was in my doctors' quarters when the phone rang. I answered it and was puzzled by so much static on the line. This had never occurred before. Then I heard a voice, very faint and so far away, calling my name as only my dad would say it! The voice, though very faint and distant, masked by so much static, was unmistakably that of my dad. I was shocked, surprised and in disbelief all at once. I managed to call out "Daddy?.... Daddy?...." and then the line went dead.

It was quite a while before I put the phone back on the hook as I felt so confused. This is the first time I am revealing this episode because now, with my understanding of the esoteric, I am not afraid to relate this incident.

The experiences I have shared confirm my belief many times over and as far as I am concerned, there is really no death as many know it. Eastern religious training has always conveyed what I believe to be the truth about death. It can not be total annihilation, just like that. Only one life time is not enough to advance ourselves, learn and experience all the lessons, return favors and pay for our mistakes, as all debts in whatever form must be repaid and at the same time all good works need to be rewarded.

This is the Universal Law. If we believe that God made us in His image, then how can we just disappear into nothing when we die? In some cases though, I believe certain souls that are not contributing much to the evolution of the whole cosmos are put into slumber, locked up in a place to be awakened only once in a millennia when the Son of God has completed his bestowal mission.

That many will say ghosts exist is another way of stating that some form of existence continues after one's death, though not the desired form of existence. Many others will still insist that ghosts do not exist. Let me relate some personal experiences with regards to this subject.

This is a logical extension to the argument of life after death. My first encounter when I was 13 years old and we were boy scouts camping. After our activities, it was time for dinner and we had to queue up for our food. It was dark by then and we were all very hungry. Suddenly one of the boys shouted out that he saw a man who looked like a Caucasian Jesuit priest which was odd considering we were in Asia! He was coming out of an abandoned old government building that happened to be near the campsite.

We knew that no one stayed in the building anymore because it was so dilapidated and had been abandoned for several years. However it was strange that the boy who saw the man was so frightened by it and this drew our attention. While we were all discussing the sighting, many of us saw the priest again, this time walking towards us and coming very near. I could see he was a tall fair skinned man, wearing the attire of a priest. As he passed by us quite closely, I even said "Good evening, Father". He just nodded his head slightly and walked back very quickly to the abandoned building and entered through one of the several doors.

Many of the boys were very disturbed by this and to prove to them it was indeed a man, although a priest has never been seen in this town before, I gathered my most brave scouts of my Panther Patrol (I was their Patrol Leader) and we went to investigate. With our flashlights and our drawn trusted scout knives, I led my bravest fellow scouts to the building!

We entered the building through the same door we had watched the man walk through earlier but found nothing inside. Then we went into all the other rooms but there was still no sign of him at all. It began to be very strange and soon the brave scouts of The Panther Patrol hurried out of the building and ran back to the campsite! We could not believe our eyes as all of us had watched him enter the abandoned building and did not see him leave. Then as we were catching our breath, suddenly some of the boys exclaimed loudly! They had seen the very same man coming out of the building once more and disappear into the night. No matter what we told our senior scouts, they never believed us. Of course we did a great job talking about this experience and no scouts ever went there to camp again.

As a doctor, I have worked in several hospitals across the nation. In one of the hospitals, one night I was the doctor on duty and it was relatively quiet but I was being constantly called to set up a drip for a patient or to get the drip running because somehow it kept on being blocked.

I was getting irritated with the nurse as she kept calling me to settle the drip problem. Then I asked the patient why he looked so dumbfounded. He then said he was puzzled because each time I corrected the problem, another man came to mess the drip up, making it blocked! However no staff ever saw this man who seemed to be able to roam about in the wards at will invisible to all except this patient. I had a restless night re-setting the drip a few more times.

Hospitals are well known to be a focus of negative forces and although I have more other supernatural experiences in other hospitals I had worked in, I shall not go into these experiences except to say I am sure that most hospital staff will have their own stories to share if you care to ask them.

The Taiwanese have a very good and therapeutic method to deal with death, especially for those who are terminally ill. They hold what is known as a 'Living funeral'. This essentially is like a conventional funeral service but the person being mourned is living and present. There are the usual eulogies, crying and hugging. The living but terminally ill person can then make his wishes known or make any announcements to his loved ones and friends. This allows them to say the things they want to say and fulfil their last wishes before it is too late and hearing their eulogies while still alive makes all the difference.

It is also important for their family and friends to express what they need to say or do and is also very fulfilling for all involved. Other types of living funerals can take the form of a last concert, tour or project to perform as a last useful act while they are still able to do so. Sometimes, this will be the only real funeral they have, since the goodbyes have already been said.

Death in many instances is sudden and leaves no time for things to be said or done. Compare this to the idea of euthanasia as practiced by some countries. It does not solve anything at all, even if it is legal. There will always be guilt and regret, with no closure for anyone. I feel that the taking of a life can never be justified, especially in cases of suicide in whatever form. The soul is very much tortured afterwards, living in the in-between world and unable to progress. Eastern religious beliefs state that one's life span is given by Heaven and if someone commits suicide, the amount of time left must still be experienced in another incarnation. Hence you can get cases of innocent young people that suddenly die for no apparent reason, leaving their family members in great distress and grief.

You can see the heavy karma ones bears if one commits suicide to escape a problem. Those who are suicide bombers bear an even heavier karma. They will discover that their place in heaven where seven beautiful virgins have been promised to them is no where to be seen. If you are able to interview those who are able to see ghosts, you will be surprised at the number of lost hungry ghosts there are around our world.

One more thing about suicide is that it tends to recur in the family, as if the demons will come again to haunt their lineage. It is best to avoid marrying into such a family as the chance of another suicide in the family is continually there.

I myself have had on at least four occasions stared death in the face, once when I joined some seasoned and professional French trekkers in the Himalayas, the other was an escape from a fiery death while in India but I wish to relate two recent episodes.

In one of my travels, I had gone to Sarawak in Borneo and to cross a river, had to jump on a little boat along with other tourists. However the boat took in water half way across the river and before I could do anything, we all went under so suddenly that I was really left in an upright position in the deep waters. Due to the shock, I found it difficult to be in a normal swimming position and was in fact struggling to keep my head above the water.

Really, it was every passenger for himself as every one was struggling. Luckily in front of me was a man and I managed to catch his shoulders and began to kick and together we were able to get to the steep river bank. We could not climb up as it was too slippery and the bottom was still very deep so we had to tread water to stay afloat. By this time the boat man had managed to climb up the bank and helped to pull many others up to safety. It was indeed a close call, and I am not sure if I saved the man in front or if he had saved me when I grabbed his shoulders and swam towards safety. All the other tourists managed to get to the bank but most lost their possessions such as expensive cameras and video camcorders.

The latest incident was when I was driving on my way to work. I felt it was a happy day. It was beautiful outside; I was in high spirits and even sang along with the radio loudly. Then a voice asked me this "What happens if you die to day?" It was odd, and I just answered that I am not frightened and have enjoyed a good life so far. I said I do not fear death as I know we are all really immortal souls. Then I had a brief feeling of "heaven" – it was so peaceful and beautiful, I never even thought of my family. I was so close to a very loving God. Before I knew it, a car came round a bend and smashed into me, head on! I did not hear any screeching of tyres, we had no time to slam on the brakes even.

The lady driver had overtaken at a corner cutting into my lane and hit me directly incredibly hard as she was accelerating to overtake a long line of cars in the morning traffic. The impact threw her car back and it landed across the road, while my car was stopped dead in its tracks. An unfortunate motorcyclist then slammed into the rear of my vehicle. I escaped with a whiplash injury and a very swollen left wrist.

The lady driver and motorcyclist were rushed to separate hospitals by the ambulances. I was trapped in the driver's seat for a few minutes. After the accident my car was in the workshop for more than eight months, the chassis needed to be changed as it was warped from the great impact. All of us survived the accident and I think it was Divine intervention that no one died. In fact I believe I had been warned about my death by a renegade monk I met a year ago but that is another long story. It shows me though that nothing is carved in stone and we can change our destiny if we change our way of thinking and choose a different path.

Since then I take my life one day at a time, living it to the fullest, doing something good whenever the opportunity arises. I give a hearty laugh if there is even the slightest humour and will not let anger and disappointment rule me. I have no time for negative thoughts or emotions any more. Now I grow more and more detached from the material and am one with the Tao.

The Buddha always taught of non-attachment to material things. Buddhist monks are supposed to own nothing but their begging bowls. This is to reduce their chances of being attached to their possessions. The reason will appear much clearer now to all who have read this chapter of why some houses are haunted - the owners were too attached to the house, their energy captured in a time/space dimension and the soul is unable to progress on its journey.

To get an idea of how tormenting this is, imagine the real world of ours and the plight of a person who is stateless. There are true cases of illegal immigrants who are caught and put into indefinite detention because their country of birth also denies their citizenship as they have "no such records" in the registers. They therefore can't be deported and have to be in limbo, with status unknown and an uncertain or no future at all as the issue can't be resolved.

Most humans have a fear of death, loss and separation and to overcome this Buddha also encouraged his disciples to meditate upon their fear in other words walk through it and unlock the secrets of the beyond. Sadhu, sadhu, sadhu!

10. Supplements – Are they required?

This is a headache to many – what to buy; which is better, do the words 'more expensive' indicate a good product? The real question to be answered is whether supplements are necessary at all? Even doctors are split in their opinions. Some argue that as long as we have a well balanced diet, we need no supplements. Others say that how ever good a diet we have, the body will do better to have some extras just in case.

Actually both can be right although the latter may have an edge over the first. My view is that we need supplements badly. This is because the quality of food that we consume these days is so bad compared to our grandfather's time, with respect to toxins, chemicals, pesticides and all sorts of other additives. The way we cook is also of great importance, with microwave cooking being the worst.

I have learned a lot about supplements mainly from my patients. They would say they had taken something and felt better and I would ask them to show me the products and soon I learned of so many brand names, companies, ingredients and am able to form my own opinion.

My humble view is that more than 95% of such products are a waste of money and precious time consuming them. To put it crudely, many people are being conned. I will discuss a few popular items just to shed some light into your understanding.

Milk is not a supplement but I am surprised that many believe in its "good for the bones" theme. First let us look at the wise animal kingdom. Young animals only rely on milk to a certain age after which they are introduced to their natural adult food whatever it may be i.e.:- grass, meat or insects. However we humans, first consume milk of another species if we are not breast fed on mother's milk. Later as adults, some still continue to consume large amounts of cow's milk.

Then another mistake is the belief that milk prevents osteoporosis. Now I can see eyes popping out with this statement. Let me explain. The calcium from milk consumed is absorbed but not in high enough amounts that the body requires. Unless you are so calcium deficient that whatever external source of calcium is taken it is absorbed. There should be no cases of osteoporosis in Western societies, which consume even more milk than Asians if the milk they consume is as good as they think.

The second point is that Asians may have lost their gut enzymes to digest milk proteins when adulthood is reached because in their culture, milk has not been a part of their normal diet. Another thing is that studies have shown milk to depress the immune system and may be a contributor to the high number of allergic issues in the population these days. Protein that comes from a cow is really the chief cause in the allergies that are developed in an exponential manner.

The melamine contamination of milk in China in 2008 caused untold miseries which was especially sad as the patients were so young. Even before this disaster occurred, I had always advised my patients against taking milk and milk products. They would raise their eyebrows and look in disbelief at this mad doctor.

Let us examine the melamine disaster in China more closely. It was greed that caused the disaster, like so many others of its kind.

The consumers were to be partly blamed, as they wanted the extra proteins in the milk and so to falsely increase the protein content, the unscrupulous businessmen devised a way to do so artificially – by adding melamine.

My point is this - once commercial production is involved and profit being the bottom line, with human greed added to the formula, the product is almost worthless. Milk is no longer milk .This concept can be extrapolated to many commercial productions.

Protein is a new word to many people and they are being misled once again. It feels like anything that is labelled to have protein in it is a good product. Do you know that foreign protein is a major cause of allergies; that too high a protein content is bad for compromised kidneys and very young children have kidneys that can be damaged by a high protein intake?

Protein digestion results in uric acid production which can lead to gouty arthritis and uric acid crystals in kidney. So are proteins a friend or a foe?

In fact the first enemy is that of the media and advertising gimmicks which the public unfortunately believe wholesomely. All the things they learn from advertisements are enough to challenge what their health professionals tell them. Funny, when truth is spoken, it seems like poison. The truth is that everything must be in moderation, the middle way - the middle path indicates absolute balance as is the yin- yang way.

The next fundamental truth is to consume anything as fresh as possible, rather than being artificially produced. Anything processed in some factory where preservative chemicals are added; which indicates possible long term storage will devalue whatever goodness it originally contained. Then the economics of business profit will further be a factor in the quality of the health product. In the end, what are we consuming?

Multivitamins – These are perhaps the best to consume as our body requires them to perform the various biochemical reactions and nearly all brands will suffice. A word of caution would be not to overdose yourself as this could mean reaching toxic levels and a strain on your kidneys. Like all supplements, it is best to stop taking them after a few months to have a 'pill-free' period for the body and for them to be re-introduced later. Continuous taking will also defeat their purpose.

Evening Primrose Oil is a favorite item of my female patients. If women are young, meaning they have not reached menopause, then the body produces enough female hormones and in physiologically correct ratios. By consuming EPO from an external source in great amounts and by the way, any amount is considered great while the body is still producing the hormones. The body is very intelligent and will eventually stop its own production or reduce it and then the lady will be reliant on an external source which may be dubious in quality due to the 'manufactured principle'. In this scenario, EPO may do more harm than good and studies indicate a high likelihood of precipitating cancer. Yes, the product labels do not tell you that. This is because EPO contains a high amount of omega 6 and when not balanced with the cancer inhibitor of omega 3, then trouble is doubled.

No wonder, with all the half truths being circulated and popularized and exploited by business enterprises, not only are people not getting better but they are getting poorer too.

Fish oils – This idea is good but only from fresh fish which has the correct ratios of the omega 3:6:9 types. Manufactured fish oils are manufactured fish oils, whatever they may say. I prefer to use the money to eat a variety of fish, which is best steamed only for 15 minutes or up to a maximum of 20 minutes. It is strange to me that people who are interested in natural foods go for capsules and tablets which are far from natural. The same arguments apply to supplements like Garlic pills. Just eat more garlic cooked along with your food. Some are just a little lazy or have no time, but often this means the food they consume is being compromised.

The list can go on and on. My intention however is not to pick at all the different supplements and discuss their pros and cons but to get to the point which is that the business men have packaged things attractively with very convincing write ups and many think they are getting something of value but really I believe they are not. Quite simply I would say that to be on the safe side it is best to go for fresh foods.

Those who think that by buying and consuming the very best supplements they are protecting themselves from many ailments may be disappointed that even after consuming so much and spending a good fortune, they are no better off. What went wrong then? Actually it is my sincere belief that many lack the art of eating.

The Art of eating the Tao way.

Taoism originated in China more than 2,000 years ago, being based on the teachings of Lao Tzu and Zhuang Zi (369 – 286 BC) with Confucius (551- 479 BC) thought as well. It emphasizes stability through harmony of the yin – yang powers of the universe. One of its philosophies is that of the 'wu wei" – 'action through inaction". Here is its philosophy on the art of eating properly.

There is actually a correct way of eating which medical science seems not to know and don't realise the importance of teaching people how to eat. In order to understand what I mean about people not eating healthily I would like to suggest that next time you eat out you observe how others eat and drink. You may see some who eat so fast like there is no tomorrow, some who eat too much while many eat the wrong type of food – oily, too many carbohydrates and sweet desserts or not enough vegetables.

This is actually very common knowledge; most every one knows deep down that we should have a healthy diet but for some reason it is not yet put into practice. Ancient Taoist masters have advised us to eat small amounts, just enough to feel half full and not gorge ourselves to the brim. This is very scientific because should we eat a very fatty meal, then the surge in cholesterols may cause a thickening of the blood and lead to chest pain (angina) or even a heart attack, especially for elderly people.

In fact it has now been proven by scientists that rats that were fed just enough lived longer than those that were over fed. It is true that the poor or homeless have meager meals; they also have lots of exercise due to no transportation of their own. Well it is also a fact that more often than not they are more healthy than the wealthy over weight who hardly walk further than the car park to their offices or condominiums.

Many are always in a hurry, rushing here and there and eating very fast, hardly chewing their food. This is a recipe for disaster. The stressful lifestyle is already having a toll on the body, what's more by swallowing food that is not chewed properly puts further stress on the digestive system, which when stressed on the whole, does not perform well. So one may eat a lot yet the body does not absorb all the supposed nutrients. In addition to this should one swallow supplements, where the quality is already suspect, then how much could really be absorbed? No wonder there are still lots of sickly people walking around.

Not only must we eat slowly, we should also chew the food well. This makes sure all nutrients are available for a proper digestion and absorption.

There is still something missing even if fresh food is eaten slowly and chewed enough. I am talking of a much higher esoteric teaching. The Tao and Zen masters ask that people refrain from useless banter, keep their minds and emotions free and just concentrate on their eating. If one is angry, sad, disturbed, then eating may do more harm than good. That is why when we were kids, our father would say "When you eat, don't talk" and he expected silence at the dinner table.

I wonder how many of you will agree with my observation – that those who eat fast are usually on the heavy side while the slow eaters are usually thin personalities. Open your eyes and observe!

The habit of saying prayers before starting a meal is indeed a good habit and also part of the Taoist way. We say thanks and invite the gods, saints and deities to partake the food first and in doing so, the foods will be blessed and when we consume such foods, they yield their nutrients to us more readily.

The same principle goes with drinking too – we are to drink fruit juices slowly, sipping a little at a time, for then the body will absorb the essence as well as the nutrients in them. The Tao master would even ask us to imagine the absorption process and this enhances the body to take up the nutrients even more. After eating they believe there should be a short period of rest, as the blood will be diverted to the gut. It is not recommended to have strenuous exercise after a meal.

To chew food well we need a good set of teeth. Those who have lost some teeth will understand how difficult it is for them to eat and really the fun of eating has been taken away. Thus dental health is important too. Animals in the wild are known to have starved to death when they have a broken jaw or tooth abscess. So I hope this is enough emphasis on dental and gum care.

In feng shui, the main door of a house is very important as good or bad qi at the doorstep determines the whole luck of the house. The main door is like the mouth of the house. This is very true for the human body, as only recently, there are studies to show how dental and gum health can be linked to heart disease. We thus see the wisdom of the ancient masters. Taoist medical philosophy is vast and would take many volumes to explain but I have shared something essential here, be aware of the front door of your house, what it represents and all that pass through it!

11. A Guide to Supplements that make the Difference

As there are so many kinds of supplements and vitamins out in the market, it is indeed a daunting task to say which are considered the best. And more are added all the time. Yet it is my opinion not to believe all that is written on the packaging. Thus with this in mind, I will try to zero in on the products that I think are value for their money and my list should not be taken as the final word nor is it exhaustive. It is just a guide, but it could also make a difference to your health.

a)   Probiotics

This is a very basic concept. The gut contains both friendly and pathogenic bacteria and the proper ratio to be kept is approximately 80: 20% respectively. However, today this ratio is largely altered in favor of the pathogenic bacteria. This comes about through antibiotic usage, poor diets, no breast feeding when as an infant or perhaps caesarean birth. The excessive use of laxatives and antacids are very common and this also results in the altered ratios form normal values. Pollution, stress and the ageing process are all contributory factors.

There are two types of friendly gut bacteria – the Lactobacillus and the Bifidobacteria Family. In the first group, it comprises of

L. acidophilus, L. bulgaricus and L. casei while the other group comprise of B bifidum, B.Longum and B. infantis. Bulgaricus DDS-14 and Acidophilus DDS-1 are the most active against pathogenic strains of E.Coli, Proteus, Pseudomonas, Staphalococcus aureus and Streptococcus.

Scientific Studies on Probiotics

1. Antibiotic action

Some side effects of antibiotics are rashes, fever, bronchial spasms, renal toxicity, nerve deafness, stomach upsets, nausea, vomiting, diarrhoea, fatigue and super infections as well as drug resistance strains emerging. However the antibiotics produced naturally by the friendly gut bacteria do not result in any uncomfortable or dangerous side effects.

In a 1977 paper, Gilliland and Speck showed that acidophilin produced by the friendly bacteria is effective against Salmonella typhimurium, Staphylococcus aureus and Clostridium perfringens. In 1984, in the paper "The role of Bifidobacteria in Enteric Infection" by Ninkaya, showed how effective it is against the dysentery organism Shigella

2. Antiviral Activity

The antibiotics have no effect on viruses and are sometimes given in the hope of preventing secondary infection by bacteria when the host immunity is depressed. So far the best way to deal with viral diseases is the production of vaccines and great strides have been taken in that direction, though there are still problems.

Antivirals are available but they are expensive and cause severe flu like side effects. Probiotics seem to be the answer. Many types of bacteria have developed ways to protect themselves against viruses other wise bacteria would have been wiped out long ago in evolution history.

The way bacteria protect themselves against viruses includes producing an acidic environment, raising the local temperature or releasing fatty acids which viruses can not tolerate.

One viricidal compound is hydrogen peroxide. In 1983, DJ Weekes published his paper "Management of Herpes simplex with Virostatic Bacterial Agent" in treating mouth ulcers due to the Herpes virus with impressive results. A paper by Klebanoff and Coombs in 1991, entitled "Viricidal Effects of L. acidophilus on HIV Type 1: Possible role in Heterosexual transmission" reported the possible role of bacteria in defeating the HIV virus. Tihole, in 1988, shares the same view when he published his work entitled "Possible Treatment of AIDS Patients with Live Lactobacteria."

3.   Anti- Cancer Activities

It is believed that environmental factors, diet, stress and genetic predisposition play a part in the cancer history. Carcinogenic substances are everywhere: arsenic, asbestos, uranium, radiation, ultraviolet rays, X- rays, tobacco and many more. Poor and wrong diets play important roles, as tumors induced in lab animals grow faster when they are fed fat-enriched diets. And 35% of all cancers are diet related.

1,2, dimethylhydrazine induced cancer of the colon in only 31% of rats that were fed with grains while it caused 83% of beef-fed rats. But when L. acidophilus was introduced into the same rats, only 40% developed the colon cancer. Thus in 1987 Fernandes, Shahani and Amer in Microbiology Reviews, listed three cancer fighting capabilities of friendly bacteria - they eliminate procarcinogenic substances before they can cause harm (nitrites), they destroy the enzymes that turn such substances into cancer causing chemicals and they directly suppress some tumor activity.

4.   Improvements to the Immune System

Our immune system is over loaded with work to combat the increasing pollutants and contaminants and this leaves us vulnerable. Thus we need all the help we can get from the friendly bacteria to free our over tired immune systems in order to deal with other more hazardous attacks.

Mice fed with L. acidophilus showed more active macrophages while human studies by Henteges in 1977, published in Cancer Research, entitled "Effect of High Beef Diets on Fecal Bacterial Flora of Human." Showed that harmful Bacteroides species increased to 100 billion per gram feces while the good Lactobacilli dropped from 10 million to 1 million per gram when high beef diets were maintained for a few months by the human volunteers. Imagine what it does to your immune system when it was shown that L. bulgaricus produced a cancer fighting agent in their cell wall called peptoglycan.

5.   Gastrointestinal Health

Food poisoning by Salmonella and dysentery by Shigella can be treated effectively with these friendly bacteria.

6.   Vaginal Infections

L. acidophilus is a normal resident in the vagina and helps to keep the fungus Candida in control. The cure rate of this bacteria against non-specific vaginitis is 95%, against Monilia is 88% and Trichomonas infections is 87%.

7.   Urinary Tract Infections

These are caused by the bowel bacteria - E. Coli, Proteus, Klebsiella or Enterobacter species and Jameson, in 1976 wrote "The Prevention of Recurrent UTI in Women." which was published in The Practitioner where he used a diet low in refined carbohydrates plus acidophilus supplements for the symptomatic relief and lifelong cure.

8.   Skin Problems

Skin care products alone will not offer great improvements in skin health when the internal environment is disregarded. Powerful antibiotics are sometimes used to combat skin problems along with steroidal-based creams. In 1964 Silver published his results "Lactobacillus for the Control of Acne" in the Journal of the Medical Society of New Jersey." He reported an 80% rate of success. However

Russian and Bulgarian doctors have used topical acidophilus pastes for decades to treat acne.

9. Baby Friendly Bacteria

This is really of concern because those who were born vaginally have a 60% rate of colonization by bifidobacteria by 6 days old while only 9% of babies born by cesarean section were so colonized. The special bacteria found in babies include B. infantis, B. bifidum, B. longum and B. breve. They are not found in adults but are as important. One disturbing trend is noted by the report from Rasic, in 1988 where he found decreasing numbers of beneficial bacteria with a corresponding increase in pathogenic ones in breastfed babies. While more than 10% have no bifidobacteria in their stools. The consequences of this shift must be viewed seriously.

10. Constipation

One of the best ways to deal with this widespread complaint is by taking lots of probiotic supplements. The bulk that makes up our stools is bacteria and increasing the number of good guys in the intestines will increase the bulk.

11. Arthritis

Ailments strongly associated with GIT problems are Crohn's Disease, Colitis and Celiac disease and the wrong bacteria may aggravate these as well as arthritis as reported by Hazenburg, in 1995 in a Scandinavian Journal of Rheumatology, 24(101): 201- 11.

12. Brain dysfunction

The overload of toxins derived from the gut and liver could be a cause of Alzheimer's disease and Parkinson's disease as reported in The Lancet, 1992; 239: 1263-64. It is reported that harmful bacteria creates such toxins. Hyperactivity in children could be due to some of these toxins from the gut. Thus a good dose of friendly bacteria goes a long way for better health.

12. Oxidation Damage

It is well known that free radicals contribute to cancers, heart disease, arthritis, scleroderma and aging. The number one site for free radical formation is in the gut, where they are created by harmful bacteria, as reported by Babbs in Free Radicals in Biology and Medicine, 1990:8(2): 191-200. Thus, friendly bacteria go to add to our antioxidant defences.

13. Fights osteoporosis

Studies by Japanese scientists (Kawakami, Ohhira, Araki, et al, 1998) from Kurushaki University showed increased bone densities in subjects over 40 years old.

14. Increased Performance by Athletes

Studies by Ohhira indicated increased Haemoglobin levels by 11.6%, and oxygen consumption increased by 23%, greatly improving endurance in marathon runners.

15. Efficacy against H. pylori

This was reported by Prof. John Lambert of Monash University who showed that the Japanese probiotic capsule was able to inhibit all strains of H. pylori and Phase 2 trials are under way. As we all may know. H. pylori is indicated as the pathogen that causes peptic ulcer disease and gastric carcinoma

As can be seen from the above discussion, if you consume the correct commercial probiotics, then you can expect prevention or cure of many diseases. Unfortunately, almost 95% of marketed probiotics are of dubious value because only live friendly bacteria make the difference. Thus their labels may say they have certain amounts of bacterial counts in their product but the percentage of live bacteria is all that is of importance. Moreover some have freeze dried bacteria and here again whether this is activated in the gut is the question. So the best way anyone can test whether bacteria will work in the body is to try and make yoghurt out of it.

In other words put some of the bacteria in milk and see if they are able to ferment the milk. Dead bacteria will not ferment milk and the more live bacteria the product has, the better the yoghurt quality.

Some companyies market probiotics derived from soil bacteria but to me soil bacteria should remain in the soil and not in the human gut. The millions and thousands of years of human evolution would have decided whether or not bacteria in the soil are beneficial.

(b)   Seaweed

The people of China, Japan and Korea have been consuming seaweed since ancient times and as for China, it was documented by Sze Teu in 600 BC and by 300 BC it was recorded as a perfect food source. The seaweeds commonly used as medicine in China are – Saccharina japonica, Sargassasum, Ecklonia kurome and Porphyra. Japan had taken the idea from China and produced the first seaweed farms in the 17th century.

There are at least 21 species of seaweed used in food preparation in Japan today. Some examples include Nori (Porphyra species), Kombu (Laminaria species) and Wakame (Undaria pinnatifida).

In the west, Ireland and Scotland have been harvesting seaweed for consumption since the 19th century. The Irish Moss which is the seaweed Chondrus crispus is recommended as a health remedy. It was used as herbal medicine by the Greeks and Romans too. In Wales, Laverbread is mainly Porphyria dioica and picked from rocks in the coastline. Many chefs are discovering how useful this is and adding them to their recipes.

Life, it is said, began in the sea as a single cell and has slowly evolved to what it is today. Thus the sea contains all the required elements to form and sustain life. Indeed seaweeds are better than any land type vegetables as far as nutritional value is concerned.

Nori has twice the amount of vitamin C as oranges, packed with beta- carotenes and rich in calcium, iron and iodine.

Arame is laden with magnesium, Potassium, calcium sodium and iodine.

Wakame is rich in iron and has 10 times more calcium than a glass of milk.

Hijiki is almost black, shredded seaweed not used in sushi or Chinese restaurants. It has high levels of arsenic and it is best not to eat Hijiki. This is the only type you need to avoid.

Saccharina and Sargassum has been used in China for cancer treatment.

Most types of seaweed are rich in vitamins A, B1, B2, B6, B12, C, E. K, pantothenic acid, folic acid and niacin. They are an important supply of nearly 60 trace elements and a source of over 12 minerals, namely sodium, potassium, calcium, magnesium, phosphorus, iron, zinc and manganese.

Some benefits attributed to seaweed consumption include – better immune system, revitalization of cardiovascular, endocrine, digestive and nervous systems, renewal of energy, lowering of cholesterol, building healthy blood and stronger bones. It protects by its anti-radiation, anti-cancer, anti-oxidant, and antibiotic effects. It is highly recommended to add some seaweed to your diet.

Commercial preparations sometimes contain too much sodium, especially the dried ones; this can cause hypertension or put a strain on the kidneys. However, as in most things in nature, it is not good to consume seaweed in large quantities daily as according to Chinese medicine, it is too 'cooling' for the blood and may cause low blood pressure, sore back, weak knees and lethargy.

(c) Enzymes

I don't understand why medical science has omitted enzymes in their repertoire. There are so many well documented biochemical books on enzymes and they are covered in Biochemistry and Science classes in the second year. Every doctor knows that enzymes are essential to life's biochemical reactions. As in many items produced by the body, like hormones, enzyme production falls as we age and so aggravates the biochemistry of life.

The real value of raw fruits vegetables and especially raw fish are their enzymes. However eating raw or uncooked food poses different dangers by way of bacteria, viruses and parasitic infections. So we always face this paradox in life on earth – good mixed with danger. This blend of yin-yang is almost always there. If enzymes are taken on an empty stomach, they are absorbed directly into the blood circulation where they help to digest the partially absorbed protein molecules unhandled by the lymphatic system so reducing allergies.

There are now many enzyme preparations available and you have to look for the one where there is value for money and not just hype. They should contain protease, papain, amylase, lipase, bromelain, cellulase and lactase.

(d) Antioxidants

I believe that if you take just the three suggestions above – probiotics, seaweed and enzymes – these are all you need as supplements. However, antioxidants these days are also very relevant and a brief discussion will be done here. You may have read some scientific articles that say antioxidants do not prevent certain cancers but I feel that we can put aside studies which are few and far between and really are these studies representing the truth?

Mostly the methodology is at a flaw, with poor sample size and choice of population but with impressive statistical analysis. The other reason could be the use of poor quality antioxidants. The basic thing is that free radicals are formed from the metabolic processes which should be eliminated by the body's own defence system but due to various factors, most remain. I do support the use of antioxidants and some will be briefly mentioned now.

1) Beta carotene for the prevention of atherosclerosis, cataracts and inhibition of various cancers.

2) Lutein for the prevention of macular degeneration.

3) Lycopene from cooked tomatoes is a defense against prostate and bladder cancers.

4) L- Methionene is a powerful liver detoxifier.

5) Gingko biloba is a brain antioxidant, it improves concentration and memory.

6) Curcumin from tumeric powder can be beneficial for colon, breast and prostate cancers.

7) Green tea has proanthocyanidins which is a natural telomerase inhibitor, meaning it inhibits cancer cell proliferation.

8) Tocotrienols from palm oil is effective against breast cancer cells.

9) Superoxide dismutase has the ability to neutralize reactive oxygen molecules.

10) L- Carnosine is good for reversing the ageing process by protecting cellular protein from attack.

11) Vit C and Vit E are well known and useful. Large doses of Vitamin C, 1,000mg can be used to prevent an impending attack of a cold.

All the above mean nothing unless you are able to source them and the best way is still eating natural foods rather than in tablet/pill form. Thus your diet should include -

a) Broccoli, brussel sprouts, spinach
b) Berries like strawberries, blueberries and raisins
c) Prunes
d) Soy products for their genistein which really is an isoflavone

(e) The Super Fiber-Husk Combination

The problem of constipation is becoming very common and needs to be corrected. All the nutritional food or supplements you swallow will do not much if your bowels are packed with feces and toxins. The clearing of the bowels is actually the most basic and important concept and is neglected by many health professionals and the general public. In fact I would suggest you clear the bowels first even before consuming any supplements.

By right, with three meals a day, we need to move the bowels three times a day but medical teaching is different – moving the bowels once a day to once in 3 or 4 days is considered acceptable, I strongly believe it is not. With a high intake of meat, this situation is made worse, as undigested protein in the gut will be putrefied by the bacteria and this process releases lots of toxic chemicals.

With constipation coming into the picture, it becomes worse still and the long transit time allows more leakage of toxic waste materials into the blood stream. Fungal over growth in the gut then ensues and causes more of the leaky gut syndrome referred to as yeast syndrome with its ill effects on health.

There are patients of mine who consume plenty of water as well as fruits and vegetables and yet they suffer from severe constipation. The treatment of constipation is then sought with the use of gut stimulants like senna, bisacodyl and even liquid paraffin. However those that take these stimulants find that they continue to require higher and higher dosages until they no longer work. The trouble is their mechanism of action, which is a gut irritant basically (for senna based products). The gut will become immune to its stimulatory effect in time, as this is a basic adaptation mechanism of the body. These types of medication are only advisable for a short while to push out the hard, impacted fecal matter.

A colonic wash out has been quite in fashion lately but I think the innovative additives that some manufacturers include such as coffee powder or herbs in the water are quite unnecessary and may be absorbed into the circulation with unknown long term effects.

In view of these short comings, I and a friend, actually a Taoist ex-monk, formulated a product I call a Super Husk – Fiber combination. It is a bulk laxative which is very mild on the gut and has good results. It is taken every morning on an empty stomach with plenty of water. Good effective results will be evident in two or three day's time. It also absorbs excess cholesterol in the gut and thus over long term usage, will bring down the blood lipids. Due to being a bulk laxative, there will be no chemical irritation on the mucosa of the gut and so it will not fail over time. The great advantage in our formulation over others is that it also serves as nutrition because of the specially blended wheat germ it contains.

It is an epidemiological fact that Africans do not have a high incidence of colon cancer because of their high fiber diet which results in a lack of constipation. However with progress and a wealthier lifestyle, I think Africans who change their traditional diet to that of a more western style will soon be having a higher rate of colonic cancer. It is always a matter of time.

It is now clear that much of our ill health originates from the poor handling of our bodily wastes. A clean and healthy inner environment is even more important than the macro environment outside. If any part of our waste elimination process is working below par, it puts a strain and extra workload on the system. In the slow process of waste elimination like constipation, it results in autointoxification via the circulatory and nervous systems. This may result in the following ailments –

Headaches Indigestion Carbuncles Diverticulosis
Backaches Bad breath Acne Fungal infections
Drowsiness Flatulence Tonsilitis Vaginal discharge
Bloating Arthritis Sciatica Bowel parasites
Fatigue Appendicitis Allergies
Depressed immune system
Asthma Boils Abdominal pain

I have kept to a minimum the best supplements I think one should try. I am sure many readers will say what about Q10, Growth Hormones and a whole list of many things they are taking and perhaps even some products of which I have not heard. Those that I have not mentioned are mainly because of the following reasons – I have not understood their potential yet, they are too expensive and with dubious claims, or some are simply a load of rubbish and not worth mentioning at all!

For the benefit of my readers, I will suggest a very potent, nutritious soup with anti-cancer potential that is so easy to make. All you need are the following ingredients – one carrot, one white radish (preferably with the leaves attached), burdock root (few slices only) and three or four shiitake mushrooms. Put them all into a pot or slow cooker with some water and make a soup. Slices of onion and black pepper are optional. Consuming this soup once or twice a week will suffice. Soup such as this is healthy, natural and easy to prepare so I would say it is well worth a try!

I believe very much in the above mentioned recipe because many years ago I was involved with a Japanese man who peddled his secret soup for cancer cure and we used part of the above ingredients. I have been gathering useful information on its effectiveness.

Let me start from the beginning of this interesting story. This Japanese man was in deep financial trouble after his business and marriage failed. He was found loitering aimlessly by my friend who then came to know of his troubles and gave him some help. Unable to live on charity form my friend, the Japanese then decided to sell his cancer curing soup he learnt form his master in Tokyo.

It seemed there was always a great demand for this soup and the queues were very long from morning till night and thus his master became wealthy. He had officials from the Imperial Palace to buy his soup and who tried to cut the long queue but were politely told to join the long line of people by the old master. The formula was only taught to seven disciples of the master and they each took an oath not to produce the soup as long as the master is still alive.

The Japanese man phoned his master to ask permission to produce this soup in Malaysia where he was currently residing to help him out of his great financial disaster and besides, he put forth the point to his master, that the promise not to produce the soup was only effective in Japan! After much persuasion he was finally granted permission.

He introduced and sold the soup to some cancer patients recommended by my friend. They must have improved because demand was getting greater and he was getting more stable financially. I was roped in by my friend to carry out a scientific documentation of its effectiveness.

Thus I got to know this unusual Japanese man and who must have liked me because one fine day, he said to me that he wanted to pass me the formula just in case he may die suddenly. I asked why me, since it was such a closely guarded secret and they had to swear an oath like a samurai. He said I was the only person who never asked for the formula from him while everybody else had wanted to pry from him the secret.

Later, and unknown to me at the time, he was cornered by some local people and we never heard from him again. Even my close friend had only sketchy details of his disappearance and was reluctant to talk about it and in fact was very scared about the whole episode and we decided to part ways for our own safety.

I have no fear with regards to this event. I trust that with positive intentions and strong belief in ourselves and the power of the universe, we will always be protected and no harm from the inside or the outside can come to us.

12. The Tao of Chinese Medicine

I have been mentioning about the Tao of this and that and I had better clarify what I mean. It will be a very difficult topic but I hope what I summarize will help in your understanding of the Tao that I speak so much about. Actually this short chapter is to possibly increase your interest in the Taoist way of thinking, thus understanding more of their minds. However, due to the complexity and great wisdom of this teaching I feel mine is a grossly inadequate explanation of the Tao Knowledge as I am merely a humble student.

Fu Hsi was credited to compiling the ancient wisdom about 5,000 years ago and he gave rise to the Ba Gua while King Wen (about 1150 BC) added his experience about 3,000 years ago. I use the I Ching divination method as invented by King Wen. The I Ching or Book of Changes escaped the great burning of the books under Shih Huang Ti (213 BC).

The three most important aspects in all that are living to the Tao are the Essence (Jing), Energy (Qi) and Spirit (Shen). Jing is the creative force of the Cosmos and is the beginning, it starts post natal and it is found in food and water. Qi is the energy that is everywhere in the Universe and in our bodies, it is found in the blood and its circulation, and in the breath. Shen is the Tao in heavens and in man is the light, thought, wisdom and intelligence.

The Philosophy of the Tao – It is a very beautiful philosophy and is as follows -

1. Purify and preserve the Essence.

2. Balance and conserve Energy

3. Cultivate Spirit; Return to the Source (God).

4. Balance and Harmony is the way of Life and is in accord with Yin – Yang balance

5. Live in accord, rather than in conflict, with Nature

I mean if we are able to follow just these five rules, what a life we would lead. The first philosophy of purifying and conserving food and water is so much needed today, more so than in the time of Lao Tzu or even earlier. Even then, Taoist masters had foreseen its basic importance. The pollution to our air, water and soil is at its worst thus far. The latest example (2009) came from a small village in Thiaroye Sur Mer of Senegal, where children were dying or maimed by lead poisoning from recycling lead of a car battery. Adults too suffered from chronic illness, many from neurological damage. The earth was being poisoned with lead over the years of extracting lead from old car batteries. What have we learned over the 2,000 years of history?

Our soil now is being artificially supported by chemical fertilizers because we are growing two or three crops per year in the same soil. In reality, the soil is still being depleted of minerals and organic matter although being given fertilizers. The result is inferior quality of produce.

No wonder we are so weak and succumb to all sorts of diseases. Lacking the proper nutrients, our immune system is vulnerable to attack.

We use energy in a myriad of ways and at the same time pollute the environment. The energy we consume (oil, petrol, coal) is dwindling and won't last forever in this form. We must find a source of renewable energy and balance and conserve it.

It is disheartening to know that many people do not believe in some form of Source, Creator, Divine, Universal life force energy these days and many who believe in God, fight among themselves, and others of a different faith.

Taoists advocate the returning to Source, not going to heaven, which is boring, in my opinion. This is the real essence of our mission – to be united in Samadhi with God Almighty while we are still on Earth.

Thought, wisdom and intelligence is part of the shen (spirit) of man and is really the mind. Thought is really very powerful as advocates of positive thinking will tell you. To control thoughts that are undesirable, meditation is one of the ways recommended.

Wisdom is not obtained from a university education but from life's experience. Intelligence is not just measured by IQ but by a host of other factors. It is only logical to improve our mind set as part of our evolution.

The Yin-Yang principle is everywhere in the Tao, it is perfect balance and harmony in action. The famous yin-yang symbol is well known the world over but only very few know what it actually means. The most important component is the small yang in the yin area and likewise the small yin in the yang area. Yin – yang is in harmony with the dual nature of this planet with its cold - hot, small - big, good - bad type of expression.

In fact we can say from the One, became two – yin and yang, then it became four, then eight and so on until we can derive the 64 hexagrams of the I Ching, which can be translated to the 64 codons of the genetic code. In fact, the I Ching is in complete agreement with the genetic code and vice versa because the 'start' codon, with adenine - thymine – guanine can be matched with the trigam for Water and the three 'stop' codons, with thymine – adenine - adenine, thymine – adenine - guanine and thymine – guanine – adenine can be matched with the trigam Mountain of the Ba Gua diagram.

It is assumed that the Yin codes are for Adenine or Guanine while the Yang codes are for Cytosine or Thymine. This is derived as follows. The I Ching said that Water is the start of Life, so we equate the Water Trigam with the 'start' codon of the genetic code. To the I Ching, Mountain symbolizes stop and stillness and so we equate it with the three known 'stop' codons and so all the 64 combinations can be worked out.

Emotions have been very well linked to organic diseases by ancient Chinese physicians and Edward Bach has studied this relationship in researching his Flower Therapy. According to the Tao excessive joy for example is linked to injuries of the heart and can scatter the spirit. Many of us have heard of some dying from a heart attack when they learned that they had won a lottery and were so ecstatic about it.

Anxiety is linked to injury of the lungs, large intestines, spleen, pancreas and stomach. Fear injures the kidneys. You too may have heard of excessive fear that causes urinary incontinence in soldiers or someone who may face death. This observation indirectly confirms what the Chinese physicians already knew.

Taoist physicians consider cancer in the body to be a disease of the blood. This is in tune with what medics know – cancer cells are spread via the blood and lymph. Therefore Taoists never advocate surgery to remove cancer since it is a blood borne disease. The Taoist thus will instead detoxify and purify the blood and then rebuild it and help to circulate it around the body through special breathing techniques like Qi Gong. This is to be followed by meditation to fortify the Four Foundations (Blood, Energy, Nourishments and Resistance) as it opens up energy channels to circulate energy.

Compare this strategy with that of modern medicine. One uses the gentle way, the other the 'Shock and Awe' technique to the body with surgery, followed by chemotherapy and or radiation. Has the use of weapons of mass destruction solved many things?

Although I have gone through Taoist initiation rites (and the experience itself was very spiritual and personal) and I follow some rules for the rest of my life, I still am lost sometimes as there is so much to digest and many new pearls of wisdom in the Tao I have yet to discover.

For one thing, I have never understood the work of Lao Tzu - his book the Tao Te Ching, written about 300BC is the first great Classic. It has bothered me and I am always striving to understand his work better. I can not call myself a Taoist without knowing a bit of Lao Tzu's work! I am no exception as I discovered later how scholars from ancient China till today will argue about the real meanings of what was written. It was not until I got the message that to read the Tao Te Ching, one must meditate on the verses written.

I actually received this insight while meditating after reading the passages and quickly writing down the inspiration I received. The whole gist of the passages brought me closer to the Tao and to try and understand what Lao Tzu had wanted us to know.

To understand a little more of Chinese medicine, let me show how the Chinese physician practicing TCM handles a case of constipation. By looking at the tongue, he will classify your blood system into over heated (dry or damp heat), neutral or cool. If the body of a tongue is a lovely pink, it is a neutral blood system. If it is red with a coating of yellow, with a dry furry texture, it indicates dry heat and if the coating is sticky or damp in appearance, this means damp heat.

In a cooled blood system, the body of the tongue is pale pink or lilac with a coating of white and moist fur. The above is counter checked with your urine type. If urine is deep yellow with scanty volume, the blood system is overheated. Clear urine or pale yellow indicates a blood system on the cool side.

In a normal blood system, the stools are well formed, moist and neither too hard nor too soft, the odor is not unpleasant. Stools that appear to be composed of undigested food are from a cooled blood system.

In over heatedness, stools are hard and dry with a bad odor. When the body has burnt out yin fluids, stools can be small and pebbly.

Now instead of medicine or herbs, the physician may prescribe you a diet according to their system of food classification into cooling, neutral and warming types.

Look at the following food classifications and you will know what types of food are best for you to solve the problem, and not just talking of "fiber".

Cooling foods include – millet, miso, soya beans, tofu, gingko, cucumber, mushrooms, spinach, coconut, lemon, prawn, squid.

Neutral foods include – beans, peas, almonds, cabbage, yam, apples, dates, figs.

Warming foods include – oats, lentils, walnuts, carrots, garlic, ginger, chicken, mutton, pork, turkey, mango, strawberries.

If your system is heaty, then cooling or neutral foods are recommended. The best foods are the neutral ones for general well being. These foods also keep your blood pH neutral, thus balancing the yin and yang forces in the body.

The use of acupuncture meridians may also be recommended to solve the issue of constipation, using the Large Intestine point 4 (hegu). This is located by bringing the thumb close to the index finger and locating the highest hump formed on the hand. Gently massage this point for one to two minutes.

Constipation may also be caused by qi stagnation in the liver and the associated complaints will be those of belching and flatulence with discomfort below the ribs. A deficient qi can cause constipation, as can deficient blood and/or kidneys which are both yang energy.

This approach is so different from western type of medicine where the treatment would probably be one of the following – enema, dulcolax tablets or suppositories and they all act as gut irritants to stimulate contraction of the bowels so as to evacuate the contents.

I wish to update you on Chinese medical thinking and this is due to the quantum leap in thinking by Dr Zhi Chen Guo who pioneered his theory entitled Body Space Medicine. It is very unique, using only fifteen types of herbs out of a few hundred in the Chinese Pharmacopeia. More than that, he based his revolutionary theories of treating the soul first and then regulating the energy circuit called Gong Zhuan.

The Tao believe that everything, every organ and every cell has a soul. The soul of the liver is called hun, that of the heart is called shen and the kidney's soul is called zhi, well known in the Tao since the time of the Yellow Emperor.

According to Dr Guo, there are two vital energy circuits in the body called Gong Zhuan , the vertical cycle and Zi Zhuan, the horizontal cycle. He also considers the space between cells and the space between organs as important passages for energy flow and must be taken into consideration for healing. His choice of herbs was based on his unique ability for soul to soul contact which helped him to choose successfully from the large amount of herbs used by Chinese herbalists so that more effective herb combination resulted.

I foresee that we will hear more and more of his unique methods of diagnosis and treatment in the years to come along with many other Taoist theories which are becoming accepted the world over and not just in China.

13. The Chakras

Before going into the chakra system, let me deal with the esoteric teachings of the human body. We have in reality, five types of bodies – the physical, ethereal, astral, mental and causal. Everyone is familiar with the physical. For the remaining four body types, no anatomical study can ever detect them.

The Ethereal body is the unseen matrix of the physical body. It is the scaffolding whereby the body builds itself up. It explains the phantom limb phenomena whereby the person whose limb has been amputated still feels pain in the missing limb for the ethereal limb still exists.

The Astral body is the vehicle whereby it allows us to feel emotions, lust, instinct and desires. Its shape takes the form of the physical body.

The Mental body is where we experience thoughts, thinking and it stores information.

The Causal body is also referred to as the higher mental body and where abstract thinking exists as well as knowledge of all past and present lifetimes. We can retrieve the information via meditation or intuition. Clairvoyants who can see past lives are able to see the information stored here.

My own past lives have been related to me by various people and the one uncanny story is that the same past life event was told to me by two independent persons who do not know each other. It seems that I was once a monk but ran away from the monastery. I wondered which Buddhist monastery could that be? As I listened to the further details, it became apparent that it was somewhere in France and I belonged to an obscure Christian sect. Apparently I did not want to stay any longer. When the past life reader told me this, I saw a flash of what I could only assume to be the past life she mentioned. There was a wooden door and I was opening it to sneak out and run away in the darkness of the night. This explained to me why for no obvious reason I simply love the French language.

Now on to the Chakras! Chakra is a Sanskrit term which means spinning wheel or vortex and they are energy centers in our body, unlike the acupuncture meridians which are energy channels. There are altogether 7 main chakras in our body but according to the shamans of South America, there are 9 main chakras, the extra two are outside the physical body. The minor chakras are the hand and foot chakras.

Understanding the Chakra system leads to the understanding of the well being of a person and in fact cleansing the chakras and untying the cords that are attached to them is a form of preventive medicine of the esoteric and highest level

Working with the chakra energy can help us understand the reasons behind people's behaviour and enables us to treat the root cause. In this way we are finding permanent solutions to problems rather than temporary suppressants. We can also learn more about ourselves and what we need to heal within.

The first, second and third chakra are known as the lower chakra, the 4th is the bridge and the fifth, sixth and seventh are the higher chakra.

Each chakra has a sound and a colour associated with it and is also linked with one of the seven endocrine glands. Every organ in the body and their functions are connected with our Chakras.

It is amazing that yogis, energy workers and healers are able to link certain health issues with a faulty chakra as will be described in brief now. It is all about balance. If one focuses attention too much on the lower chakra without any apparent reason ones sexual or survival instincts may become activated and depending upon how balanced a person is this may lead to undesirable behaviour in some people.

The 1st Chakra (Muladhara) is at the base of spine, the seed of the coiled Kundalini. It is represented by a circle with four lotus petals. It is known as the Root Chakra and is linked to the adrenal glands, musical note C and to the colour red. When one is balanced the red in the Root Chakra indicates passion, vitality and life! When out of balance red signifies anger and fire. This chakra is concerned with our roots and basic survival instincts which include money, food and shelter.

The health problems related to the Root Chakra are for example sciatica, varicose veins, low back pain and rectal tumours or cancer. Other ailments manifested here are nephritis, kidney stones, cystitis and low blood pressure. It houses the kundalini.

In a worst case scenario when one is really off centre and not rooted, the kundalini fire manifests as severe aggression and this is why some people resort to hostile behaviour and terrorism which can result in global violence. They feel they have to fight to survive and hold on to their roots.. Humans who have an energy imbalance in this area will instinctively want to satisfy their basic need which is self preservation at all costs. They don't know that what they actually require is to balance their inner energy centre to achieve this result. A majority of the populace is still at this level.

In order to balance the energy here is to work on the emotional issues related, such as fears, insecurities and worries relating to survival. A recommended therapy for imbalance in the root chakra is to ground self by walking barefoot in nature, dancing and anything which will allow a person to feel safe etc.

The 2nd Chakra (Svadhisthana) is located in the lower abdomen or at the hypogastric pluxus of nerves. Mystics see it as a circle with six red petals. It is known as the Sacral Chakra and is associated with the sex glands, the musical note D and the colour orange. When we are in alignment orange signifies creativity, imagination, sensuality, creation, children and the inner child. It is connected to the astral plane.

To give an example of colour, its meaning and the impact and significance it has on us take Holland. It is famous for the colour orange. It is also famous for being very sexually liberal. The Dutch are intrinsically open minded and sexually free without inhibition which is what the colour orange basically represents - sensuality, sexuality and creation.

If one is off balance in this area it can mean sexual dysfunction, sexual addiction, possessiveness, jealousy reproductive disorders, fibroids, allergies, skin problems, low back pain, haemorrhoids and urinary system ailments.. Also connected with this chakra system are cancer of reproductive organs, herpes and genital warts.

In order to realign or prevent health problems here we must allow freedom of expression and imagination, we must nurture the inner child within us all and have a balanced sex life. The best therapy for imbalance of the Sacral Chakra is anything sensual for example a massage or spa treatment; anything creative such as painting and playing, in other words letting the inner child out. A good form of exercise here would be Yoga or belly dancing!

The 3rd Chakra (Manipura) is at the solar plexus, roughly two inches above the navel and is known as the Solar Plexus Chakra. It is depicted as a circle with ten blue petals, representing the ten dimensions of space science is yet to confirm. This Chakra is associated with the pancreas and liver glands, the musical note E and the colour yellow. This is the colour that represents our being and mental clarity. The Solar Plexus Chakra holds the energy of the will to make things happen, it is our ego and power centre, the seat of emotion and it is the last place for us to have feelings based on ego before crossing the bridge to the higher Chakra. It is the gut where we use instinct and feel inner resistance as we are learning to let go of the ego and therefore a multitude of emotions and power struggles are represented here. It is where we want to show our authority and to feel important, before we move on to the heart and know that we are loved, it is here we try to prove our worth. It is also a centre for psychic energies.

When the energies in the Solar Plexus Chakra are balanced we have a healthy relationship with power, it doesn't go to the head and we are confident, yet humble and not overly emotional, usually financially successful, powerful and secure. If people are out of alignment here they are often very stressed. They have a huge ego, tend to be over confident and very sensitive, stubborn, boastful, proud and full of insecurities, self loathing, worries and fears. To be well balanced here is to have a sunny disposition and ready to evolve to higher states of consciousness.

Health issues related to this chakra are problems of gastrointestinal tract, anorexia nervosa, arthritis, liver problems, gall stones and pancreatitis/diabetes. Many nervous break downs are due to energy dispersion from this chakra. All mass hysteria originates from here.

In order to heal or prevent health issues in this area is to work on self empowerment and build self esteem, confidence and self respect. It is recommended to focus on inner peace by using relaxation and breathing techniques.

The 4th Chakra (Anahata) is at the cardiac or heart area and known as the Heart Chakra, the beautiful bridge to higher levels of consciousness when one opens the heart. It is represented by a circle with twelve petals and within this is an eight petaled lotus, representing the eight emotions. The heart Chakra is the connection joining ego love to higher love and beyond, it is associated with the colour pink for romantic love and green for universal love. The Heart Chakra is also linked with the musical note F and the thymus gland.

It represents love and compassion and when one is in alignment he or she is very loving, compassionate, joyful, filled with appreciation, self love and love for the whole; flowing easily through life with a very light vibration attracting love and happiness towards them. The higher part of the bridge represents unconditional and universal love without limitation. Blockages here can result in neediness, loneliness, holding grudges, revengeful and unkindness due to feeling unloved which can lead to heart failure, heart attack, asthma, allergies, lung cancer, breast cancer and upper shoulder back pains. AIDS, scleroderma, lupus and rheumatoid arthritis are other manifestations of a blocked fourth chakra.

Recommended ways to keep the Heart Chakra energies in balance are emotional exercises that open the heart such as learning to give and receive equally, appreciation and self acceptance. If one works on wholeness, self empowerment and self sufficiency he or she will become closer to their Inner Being who is Love and will realise that all the love you need is within yourself. Love from the outside is just an added bonus but he or she will not be able to receive it if they cannot first receive from themselves.

The 5th Chakra (Vishuddha) is also known as the throat chakra. In Tantric art, it has a circle with sixteen petals and is a centre of psychic dreams. The Throat Chakra holds the energies of the thyroid gland and shares the vibration of the musical note G and the colour blue. Blue is known as the colour for loyalty, truth, courage, protection and spiritual wisdom.

Situated at the throat it is thus associated with communication and expression and when a person is balanced in this area he or she is open and converses clearly. People whose energy is in equilibrium here are not afraid to speak their truth and they communicate with much wisdom. When out of alignment health issues related to this chakra are speech problems like stuttering, thyroid problems, throat and mouth ulcers, chronic sore throat and depression. Often when one has a sore throat or cough, those in the know will ask them what they are suppressing and are afraid to express.

The Throat Chakra is the first of the higher Chakra and therefore represents spiritual truth and being oneself without fear. When ones words are cutting and sharp tongued he or she has not balanced their energy in the Heart nor the Throat Chakra and may find mouth ulcers developing. Those who do not speak with truth are very out of alignment and totally off track. They are unable to face themselves and have much work to do on the lower Chakra before even beginning to express who they think they are.

To keep the 5th Chakra energies in balance is to make sure that the words that come out of your mouth represent how you feel inside. One must not hold or bite ones tongue but express freely. Singing is a really good way to convey what is in your heart and when you sing so too do your cells. It is important to sing happy songs and if you find yourself listening to sad music that makes you cry it is your inner self craving to heal. The music you listen to also reflects whether you are totally balanced in this area.

There may be times you feel like screaming, you must always listen to yourself and communicate with your own body, mind and soul too. Listening is another important attribute of this Chakra. Communication with your Inner Self is the highest level of the Throat Chakra.

The 6th Chakra (Ajna) is centre for visualization and insight. It is at the point between the eyebrows, the so called Third Eye Chakra. The Ida, Pingala and Sushumna energy channels meet at this point. In acupuncture, there is the Governor Meridian which has correspondence with the Sushumna channel. Ida is to the left of the spinal channel and represents the female (of) Yin energy while Pingala is to the right and is the male Yang energy.

The Third Eye Chakra is associated with the pituitary gland, the musical note A and the colour Indigo. It is the energy centre for intuition and inner connection. It is a higher energy which no longer needs to communicate through words but through thoughts and feelings.

When we are balanced in this area we begin to become more intuitive and find much synchronicity. We understand more clearly the bigger picture of life and see far beyond the vision of the eyes. When all our Chakra are in balance our vibration becomes light and we can manifest the things we desire very quickly as we find doors opening for us. The eyes are like the windows to our soul and with the third eye awakened we can see inside.

When this area is out of balance people are very sceptic and unimaginative. Some have tunnel vision which becomes almost like a pressure of energy trying to break through the blinkers and open ones eyes. Medical problems associated here are headaches; migraine and eye problems are characteristic including both long and short sightedness, neurological disorders, blindness, deafness, seizures and sinus problems.

The Third Eye Chakra communicates with both throat and heart energies. Exercises to keep the energies in this area balanced and in tune are visualisation techniques, meditation, trusting and developing the intuition. It's about thinking not only of oneself but of unity and a worldly connection with all. To be balanced here is to trust you are not alone and to know there is a bigger picture and that everything that happens in life is for our spiritual growth. The Third Eye Chakra is in perfect alignment when we have a deep and loving connection within.

The 7th Chakra (Sahasrara) is associated with free will and divine wisdom. It is situated at the top of the head and yogis believe it to be the seat of the soul. It is depicted as a thousand petaled chakra. This is known as the Crown Chakra and is linked to the musical note B, the colour violet and the pineal gland otherwise known as the master cell in the brain.

This chakra is our connection to all that is and the higher realms. It is the chakra of enlightenment, oneness, harmony and knowing. The Crown Chakra connects us to infinite wisdom and Universal love and light.

When we are in balance and of a light vibration we connect through the Crown to the higher realms of unconditional love and Source energy. It is the portal through which energy enters our bodies.

When we are out of balance we can feel separation, closed in, suffocated, unable to learn and anti social. The health problems related to this chakra are paralysis, bone cancer and genetic disorders.

To maintain balanced energy here is to maintain balanced energy through all the Chakra by meditating, visualising and spending time in a joyful and loving state knowing that we are all one and never alone or separate. To experience communion with ourselves is to experience spiritual union with Source energy, as above so below.

The first five chakras are connected with the five elements. If the desires for survival are not fulfilled, one takes birth after birth as a human. If desires of the second chakra are not met, one dwells in the astral plane after death and after sometime, chooses rebirth to fulfil the desire. This is the relationship between chakras, rebirth and spirituality.

You will notice that most of the diseases originating from Chakra bodies are those that medical science has not much information to offer. This is not a coincidence I tell you. To me, this is an indirect proof that the root cause was not dealt with by those conducting scientific studies. Western medicine is good at figuring out how to bring relief of symptoms and these are seen to act fast sometimes but they never find an actual cure. They merely offer something that suppresses the symptoms which gives one a false sense of security until the issue at hand squeezes out in another way and thus the relief is only temporary. I call this way of dealing with things a big bluff.

When I finished my medical school training, I thought I knew everything that needed to be known to heal my patients but I was wrong. I felt like a fool. I remember being so greatly embarrassed one day when an old Chinese man from a poor background, asked me to solve his rather insurmountable medical problems and I remember he had a big dilemma and he believed me whole heartedly when I said I could, just to give him hope.

Actually there wasn't much I could do but he made me feel deep inside that I must improve my knowledge. I felt an esoteric connection with this stranger who I never saw again but always remember. He played a significant role in helping me expand; I still remember his face because he has made a deep impression on me. He was like a messenger from the Universe and I will always be grateful to him. When we are aware of these Earth Angels that come into our lives no matter how subtle they seem at first they can help open many doors that we only know exist because they remind us to look for them.

I decided to do all I could to receive more knowledge and improve myself so that with the extra know how, I was sure I could do more. Again I was wrong, my medical quest took me to a Diploma, Fellowship and Masters and yet I still felt so helpless. That was when my search led me to choose another road in my quest for more knowledge and I discovered so many amazing less travelled but more fulfilling pathways I never would have found if I hadn't always strived for growth.

In my search of knowledge and truth, my thinking began to change. As I have mentioned before it was at this time I noticed my medical colleagues and friends thinking so highly of themselves as having superior knowledge and quite a few even looked down at the uneducated. I was aghast when one of my close friends from school days refused my invitation to eat at a cheap place where the food was really good. We used to eat there when we were school boys, but here he was saying he could not be seen in such places anymore as his community would look down upon him.

I had even more such encounters with many other colleagues over the years so now I prefer my own company and whenever I attend any medical meetings I do my own thing and keep pretty much to myself. I don't feel it necessary to stay back for long after I have gained whatever knowledge I can from the meeting.

I have nothing against these people and the real reason that I am unable to remain in their circle is the energy. We are no longer a match, our vibrations do not resonate and quite simply we do not attract each other's company. I feel it hurts my chakras and aura to be in an environment where there is a resistance between us and not a natural flow.

Before changing my vibrational energy, I used to be able to go to a casino to look around and see how people gamble. However now, things are different. One time not too long ago I accompanied some friends to a casino and found that my perspective had completely changed. I saw it like a scene in hell – the people so mesmerized in their gambling with all sorts of energy that was not like mine. I could feel the greed, the anger, the disappointment and the tension in the air. I saw blackish clouds over most people; they looked like zombies, the walking dead. More than this, I felt so uncomfortable in my heart that I felt nausea and spells of dizziness.

The moment I walked out of the casino, I recovered like magic. This happened two or three times and I knew the energy was so bad and negative in the casino that I will never walk into one again. No wonder, one of the qigong masters had once said the energy of the whole locality where the casino stood had bad qi. This was the reason he refused to go there for a retreat although it has got excellent facilities and cool weather as it is at the top of a mountain range.

I once went to a temple and when I was just outside its doors, I was puzzled with the mixed emotions that suddenly engulfed me and could even "see' many souls clamoring around me in my mind's eye. It is true that at places of worship, lost souls in limbo will gather trying to receive merits to enhance their standing. This also proves to me what my feng shui masters taught us, that temples and places of worship are not giving out as much good energy as most would think.

Through the chakra we are blessed with a number of energy vortexes to help us interpret signals around us and assist in guiding us in directions we are aligned with. If we feel discomfort in a certain area of our body or have some physical disease these are signs showing us which areas need to be worked on. For example if we have lower back pain, we know this is related to the root chakra and can therefore check whether we are feeling insecure about money or threatened in some way. Once we work through these emotions the pain is usually relieved. If we leave it for too long without being aware of the indicators we will find they grow larger until we cannot help but notice them.

Stress of any kind, can result in our chakra being out of balance which can eventually lead to disease. When we balance these energy centres we can heal our diseases. Better still is to be proactive and always keep our Chakra finely tuned so we can remain healthy physically, emotionally, mentally and spiritually. We are blessed to have so many clues and indicators guiding us always in looking after our health wholesomely.

14. Strange Illness caused by the Unknown

This will be a most controversial chapter as I am going to deal with forces some may not accept, demanding proof but nevertheless I need to share my experiences with those who will listen. By the word unknown here I do not mean the medical equivalent of "idiopathic" or "fever of unknown origin". In medical jargon, these words inform the doctors that so far, all tests reveal nothing as a cause which perhaps will be revealed at a later date when more tests are conducted.

However what I am saying here is that there is absolutely no medical cause to be discovered now or later. Doctors per se are trained to have logical and scientific minds and so folk lore, old wives tales and grandmother's stories are never accepted. Well, I include these here as fodder for thought.

Let me share some of my personal experiences to let you know what I mean. Of course you must form your own opinions as I too have formed mine.

The first event I would like to share is with regards to a friend who phoned me to say that he was having difficulty in breathing. I told him to go to the nearest hospital and not any clinic. However this chap drove all the way to see me and I did all the necessary tests like an ECG for the heart and blood tests along with a detailed physical examination and found nothing wrong. I reassured him that there was nothing physically wrong with him.

He then proceeded to give me the most interesting feed back. He said that it is funny that almost every year he would go through a similar experience and this included being admitted to hospital for observation. Each time this yearly event has occurred it was on the 7th Lunar month of the Chinese calendar. This is the Hungry Ghost month observed by the Chinese and is a most feared month as these ghosts are allowed to roam and mingle freely with humans for the entire month.

I laughed at him and said it was only a coincidence. When I checked his records for the last year, indeed he had a similar attack of chest pains with difficulty in breathing around the same time, however he hadn't mentioned to me about his ghost month syndrome at that point as we had just recently met. Unfortunately I lost touch with this interesting character shortly after this.

I did not believe in the ghost month at that time until my own nurse had a very prolonged illness that I was not able to cure. She complained of fever, sinusitis, headaches, gastric upsets, vomiting, nausea and insomnia with difficulty in breathing at night. I was really stumped by the fact that all the medications I gave her had not solved the problems. This really bothered me as she was suffering so much,

I decided to refer her to an ENT consultant to have a look at her sinusitis. The next day, she came to work more bright and cheerful and full of energy. What an amazing recovery, I thought. She then revealed to me that she had gone to see a temple medium instead who had given her some holy drink to swallow and in the next instant, she felt so much better and relieved!

She was told that she had annoyed a wandering ghost and so was taught a lesson. It was again the ghost month of the Chinese. This was getting too much, but because it involved my own nurse whom I see every day and who was under my care, it made me wonder more about this ghost month thing. The funny part was that she had these funny illnesses almost every ghost month although she was very careful about her health. In her case, I now think that she was quite vulnerable because she has an increased sixth sense and so a very easy prey to spirit influences.

Very recently, just prior to the completion of this book, I had another strange case. A distressed mother brought her 6 year old son to see me with the complaint that he kept vomiting after every attempt of food or water consumed in the last 5 days.

She had taken her son to see two different doctors who gave treatment but there was no response. I had to do something for the child and I used all my experience and knowledge to look for a possible pathology indication but found none. It was puzzling and I noticed also he had a very funny, awkward gait, which the mother denied he had prior to this complaint.

I asked the mother to take the boy to see a temple medium and indeed she took him that very day and the medium achieved what we doctors could not – he was well that very moment after some prayers and holy water. This again happened during the Ghost month and the medium told the woman not to take her son out at night during this time. I had nearly admitted him to hospital a few hours earlier.

Now I began to be more observant during the ghost months and indeed I noticed that there are always increased incidents of motor vehicle accidents on the road during this time. I find I will travel the same roads all year and will not see any accidents on them except during ghost months.

Many Chinese patients are reluctant to undergo surgical operations during this time if they can help it. In the hospital that I am attached to, even the nurses will comment that elective surgical cases are so much less during the said month. It is of course of great taboo to hold important occasions like weddings and the opening of new businesses throughout this special month, and this every Chinese person will know.

In the town where I stay, it is noticeable that for the duration of the Hungry Ghost month, there are fewer people on the roads at night as many prefer to stay in doors if they have nothing important to do. Thus businesses in general are quite affected. I too tend to avoid a very winding and isolated road as I have noticed people seem more accident prone at this period.

This Ghost Month is a very important religious celebration in the Chinese calendar for the people of George Town, Penang. It is a month long period of prayers for the departed. Communities in different localities will pool their resources and pray to the King of Hades with lavish offerings and a stage show. Lately a majority of these stage shows feature young and scantily dressed sexy singers. However, Chinese Operas are still being staged. These celebrations are a great tourist attraction.

I have another incident I would like to relate but before I begin I would say that qualified doctors all know what is considered 'normal' anatomy, physiology and biochemistry in order to understand what are deemed abnormal and diseased states.

Over the years, I have developed a bit of psychic ability perhaps due to my meditation. One day, a patient was brought by a woman relative who asked me to check her. Those were her only instructions. As I was taking the history of the patient and hadn't even done any physical examination yet, I noticed that I had a very uncomfortable feeling which was getting stronger and stronger.

As I had prior experience of such a feeling in another episode, I knew at once what it meant. I realized that she was being possessed by some spirits and at once told the relative to take her to an appropriate place where she would be helped as it was not a medical case. The relative was surprised at my conclusion because she knew there was something odd about the way she acted and I confirmed her suspicions.

The story was then revealed to me. This lady was of perfectly sound mental state and had gone to London to meet up with her husband who was working there. She began to exhibit strange behavior after being there a few months. She had to be taken back to her home town accompanied by her sister as the doctors there could find nothing medically wrong with her and she was getting worse.

The relative then asked me where to take her as they had no idea. Since she had accepted my diagnosis, I thought then I could help her as I was in contact with a medium. I phoned the medium and he was available and I got another friend to accompany them as they didn't know the way to the temple.

What ensued was incredible. The lady, who I felt was possessed, had been quiet all this while, suddenly began to act very aggressively and struggled to get out of the car. It was lucky my friend was there and he was able to subdue the woman and contain her.

Later I found out that at the temple, the woman became even more violent and trance-like and then she fainted. My friend the medium went to work immediately to exorcise her. It seems that what followed was quite a battle. My explanation is that while in London, she had been possessed by a troubled spirit. I last heard that my medium friend was able to solve her problem and she was back to normal again.

My next case is equally interesting. A man brought his wife to see me for an ordinary cough. Then upon history taking, I discovered that she had seen lots of doctors all over town for various ailments until they had nearly exhausted their funds. I asked if they had engaged a feng shui master to check the energies of their house. They were very surprised but answered my question by saying that yes they had engaged not one but two and both had said there was nothing wrong with the house. I said anyway if they wanted another opinion

I would gladly do it for them as I thought her problems were feng shui related.

Not too long afterwards, I received a call from the husband who said they were willing to give it another go as they had nothing more to lose anyway. Both husband and wife were at their wits end. So I fixed an appointment. On my way there on that appointed day, I accidentally knocked into another car as I was parking although I was very careful. As there was no visible damage to both my car and the other parked and stationary car, I proceeded to the house and did the preliminary work of taking directions and noting the floor plan.

I left and said that I will take a few days to come up with my analysis. On my way back I became exceptionally sleepy and yawned several times. Then, at the junction of a road, we had to stop at the red lights and I fell asleep, allowing my car to slide slowly forward and hit the car in front! Again, there was no visible damage, the driver did not make a fuss and the lights turned green and off we went. I thought all these little incidents were very odd.

I finished my analysis and was very surprised at what conclusions I had come up with – most importantly was that I felt they really had to move out of the house for their safety! I had never so far asked for this drastic action in my many other cases. I determined that there would be impending death in the house or that it had already occurred. Moreover they would be involved in many accidents in the future. I made a quick appointment to see the couple. When I arrived with my printed report, the husband was out and I was told he would return shortly as he had just been in a minor accident. I very nearly fainted!

When the husband came back, with dressings and bruises, I gave my report. They listened without saying a word. When I had finished, the man said that the two other feng shui masters they had engaged never said any of the things that I had mentioned and above that, they had been assured that their problems were solvable by following their instructions. I told them I wasn't able to fight the great forces (the shar qi) that were attacking their place and also I deemed it life threatening if they continued to stay on. They confided that the wife had recently suffered a miscarriage. In feng shui terms, this is already a death. It did not take them long to decide to move to another place.

They in fact asked me to look at their new place to check it out and I was glad to do so since I had noticed that sometimes, no matter where people run, unless they work on their issues they will choose a house with the same bad feng shui. This is their karma. This couple moved into the new place and after 2 months, they were very happy because all the ailments that were nagging the wife had disappeared without using any antibiotics, pain killers or steroids. Not a tablet was swallowed. In fact, her health improved greatly. The couple must have done some serious reflection and inner work and understood the importance of my guidance and ever since then, they always seek my advice, both medical and other.

Thinking back on this case, I now know the reason why I had the small accidents when I was going to their evil house and after I left. The evil forces were giving me a warning not to meddle with their plans. It became clear to me that if I were to continue with this kind of work, I would need some kind of protection, hence the talismans I now wear around my neck.

I am going to relate a story about my dear old mother, Nuah Gaik Kin, also affectionately known as NGK. At one time, she was having quite frequent incidents of upset stomach and I treated her as a case of mild food poisoning but there was not much response. Then after some time it would return and this happened over and over again, on each occasion I would start the standard anti-diarrhea treatment thinking she perhaps had an irritable bowel. I noticed however that it seemed to be getting worse and it pained me very much to see her suffer. She was already 87 years old and seldom would trouble me with any complaints.

When she did not get better, I decided to do a complete investigation to rule out sinister problems, especially that of any colonic growths.

All tests came back negative. Although it was a huge relief there was still no diagnosis. My brother, Hock Lye, himself a medical consultant also gave his input but we could not solve this case and the issue that kept coming back to bother her. I was troubled, as were all my siblings, from Annie Yeoh in Singapore to Milly Yeoh in Sydney. I was under pressure to solve the problem for mom.

I finally decided to ask one of my feng shui masters from Hong Kong his opinion and he advised me to just shift the position of the table fan that mom used . He actually chided me for not diagnosing it myself as it was so clear cut to him. After this advice, mother improved tremendously with fewer attacks! However, there were still some minor incidents off and on.

'Now what!' I thought and spent much time in deep contemplation and one day I said I had better open my feng shui eyes again! And viola! I spotted the cause.

You see, I had a special water feature in the front part of my house that is for feng shui purposes. The placement of the water feature was well calculated to be in a strategic position. Now, I noticed that the water pipe was directed at my mother's bed and this was afflicting her. I quickly removed the water feature – my thought was forget about obtaining wealth, health is more important.

It was like magic, within a week, she had no more attacks. I was exhilarated. Unknowingly, I had caused mom some problems but luckily I was able to solve the quandary. I had always been wary of playing with water cures in the feng shui sense as I know it to be a double edged sword. This was a good lesson. Mom NGK passed on two years later when she was 89 years old while she was sleeping, and I was able to perform a last offering to her by easing her onward journey with Reiki and Buddhist prayers.

I know, at least on three occasions, I have saved my mother's life by my timely and swift action. This time, I just had to let her go to Buddha Land. It was very lucky too that my sisters from abroad were both at home and who alerted me as I was staying some 7 km away. I rushed as soon as I got news that mom NGK was gasping and breathing her last. I prayed to God to allow me enough time to reach mom and I did. She passed on peacefully within 3 minutes of my arrival. I knew the meaning; she had waited for me to come before she was willing to go.

The bright morning suddenly turned cloudy and even a few drops of rain hit the awning, and then it stopped. This was another sign from Mother Nature. You see, mom was able to ask for good weather and she always got it. When she flew to Australia, she was afraid of the winter and prayed for a mild one. The moment she left Australia, and after my sister was about to leave the airport, the weather suddenly turned cold and remained so until winter was over, and this happened every time she went there.

Back here, when the rain storms came and she knew I was about to come home, she would pray for the rain to stop, and I would at times wonder how suddenly the storm was down to a drizzle and back to a storm the moment I reached home. Yes, mom would talk to nature. She appreciated the birds that sang in the trees and said out loud 'Oh, birdie, I like your song." I noticed that almost the same time every day, the same birds would sing. Sometimes, mom would say "Birdie, sing for me." Then a bird would somewhere in the trees, just chirp. I was witness to this beautiful connection and when mom passed on, I noticed there were no more birds singing from the trees. I called to the birds to sing, but there was no response.

This next case although was not a peculiar health problem, was also solved by my use of feng shui. A relative of mine had two sons that were driving each other and their parents crazy. They were at logger heads with each other, always quarrelling and generally becoming uncontrollable. It was only a matter of time before they were about to go for the jugular, as they say.

These boys were growing physically bigger and stronger too. Their father had wanted me to refer the trouble maker to a psychiatrist or psychologist. I thought that was an extreme solution and besides, I have never believed in all the drugs or medications used by any psychiatrist. I think, of all the branches in medicine, psychiatry to me is the maddest of all. Medical science as such really does not understand the mind, although the brain is just an anatomical component. Adjusting the level of dopamine or other neurotransmitters does not constitute a cure to me.

Anyway I told them I would not refer the boy to a psychiatrist as yet until I attempted to solve the problem my way. I made a special trip to their house in Kuala Lumpur, about 350 km from where I was staying, to look into the energy aspect of their house. I made another trip when I had calculated and understood the distribution of energy. I discovered that the room the boys were staying in had the worst energy and may have contributed to their quarrelling nature and disobedience. Even at school, the teachers were having a headache as the younger boy had become very aggressive and was generally quite a problem with regards to discipline.

I had suggested that they move out of the room and in to another one. That was not a problem, the father explained but he asked if other people would be able to stay in that room? This was because one of his relatives, Seng, was sharing the room with the boys. I said no one should stay in that room as it had such negative energy. He took my advice.

There was no news from them for a few months and I wondered if my suggestions had worked. I could not wait any longer for his phone call so I called my cousin up. What he told me even knocked me off my feet. He said there were far less quarrels between his two sons and their mother. Not only that, even the teacher noticed the change in the younger boy, who no longer caused trouble in the class but also was doing his home work.

However, Seng, had benefited the most since being kicked out of the room and put in the hall way. Seng had suffered three motor vehicular accidents while he was still in the room and also lost his money and job. After being pushed out, his luck became tremendous - he had found a job and even won a small amount of money in the betting of numbers!

Here is another story of case that I felt was also weird and it was a patient of mine who as a last resort came to consult me after all the specialists in town could not help her. She complained of having a sensation of something around her neck that caused her to feel constricted and with burning pain.

In my examination of her neck region, I could find nothing wrong. She told me that she even had a biopsy done and it turned out normal. She really was at her wits end. I then suggested that she come back later as I would first consult a psychic friend of mine to investigate as I suspected some deep issues within her psyche.

My friend investigated and came back with this story. In her past life, she was a military man in some European country and while on sentry duty, had accidentally slipped and fallen through the wooden floor. The string attached to his rifle caught round his neck and he had a horrible death due to accidental hanging.

This accounted for the trauma that had resulted in her having this peculiar burning sensation around her neck region. During her next visit to me, I related to her what the psychic had told me and she just looked shocked. Then she said that at the last consultation with me I had given her the idea to investigate it herself. She had consulted a priest in the temple who also told her it was a past life trauma and for her to do certain prayers to solve the problem. She had felt rather sceptical at first but now after hearing what I had told her, she said she would proceed with the special prayers. I never heard from her again and I presume finally her problem was solved.

My last story to relate here is about our famous feng shui Grandmaster, a jovial old man who was so energetic at his age it was hard to keep up with him, his stamina made young people feel they should be more active! He travelled all over the world to teach as well as do feng shui audits. One day, word was out that Grandmaster was mysteriously not contactable. It sent shivers down every spine of his loyal students. No one knew where he was or what had happened. We were all stumped.

Finally, after some time, we were called to have dinner with him, the inner circle students. Usually we adjourned to a restaurant and settled in a corner with a screen to stop the general public from seeing us, as Grandmaster being so well known, did not want people to spoil this meeting with his students. I heard what he said from a friend as I missed the dinner due to work commitments.

He was indeed very sick while in Romania. His strength was slowly being drained from him and he became weaker. This was unusual, as he practiced qigong and charged himself up often, however this time it did not work that well. It got so bad that he was admitted to hospital in Romania. He was very pale and the doctors there did a range of tests and the only positive finding was the severe anemia but they could not determine where the bleeding was from. He had blood transfusions but still grew weaker. The situation was really critical. The doctors were at their wits end.

Unknown to the doctors or to his aides there, Grandmaster was fighting a psychic war with a most evil entity he picked up somewhere in Romania. It was a battle royal indeed. If grandmaster won, he would get his life back. There was no question of losing! No one was able to fight this battle for him. In the end, grandmaster was able to subdue this entity and win him over and ever since, they have become very good friends. Grandmaster had the cheek to invite this entity to follow him to Malaysia!

It is of great concern to me that these days we are seeing more cases of black magic and also of body possessions by wayward spirits. My observations proved correct by a recent report from an Islamic medical practitioner who specializes in removing charms and witchcraft. Of the reported 1,200 students from my country screened by him in Cairo, he claimed that 153 were affected by spirits (12.75%)

and 114 by black magic (9.5%). Back in Malaysia, a well known ghost buster screened more than 20,000 people over seven years and found a rate of 4% being charmed by black magic. Mass hysteria is a rather common affliction among factory workers in Malaysia and most likely to be precipitated by spirits.

Medical examination of those affected by spirits and black magic will reveal nothing abnormal in almost all cases. However these victims do suffer some ailments or a change in behavior.

It is also true that as we have a deeper connection within we can also have a connection with the most loving energy and guidance and be in spiritual union with all things just as my mother felt with the birds and environment. We can all have this bond, all we need do to have it is believe we can and be 'Love'.

As you can see that in cases where I am not able to help the patients of mine, especially those with peculiar ailments, I would refer them to the relevant authorities, be they ghost busters or people with other special gifts. Now I wish to add a further dimension – that of the gods that heal.

In most of the Taoist communities especially in Asia, there are many temples dedicated to deities that are revered by their followers. Most of these deities were legendary figures; some were recorded in Chinese history. Famous generals were 'deitified' and prayed to for their blessings of safety, protection and courage, like that of Kuan Kong of the Three Kingdoms era.

Famous physicians were also made deities and prayed to for their guidance in healing all sorts of ailments. Some of the physicians extraordinaire are described below.

Bian Que, also known as Pien Ch'iao (circa 500BC) was an excellent diagnostician and it was he who first used pulse diagnosis which is still being used by TCM practitioners of today.

Shen Nong is known as the Father of Chinese Medicine, introduced acupuncture while Chong Chung-Ching (168-196AD) of Han Dynasty is known as the Hippocrates of China.

A book written by Zhang Zhongjing (150-219) on febrile illnesses is still being referred to by modern day TCM physicians.

The greatest herbalist of China was Li Shih-Chen (1518-1593) of the Ming period (1368-1644) who took 27 years to write his pharmacopoeia, which is still being referred by modern day TCM herbalists.

Not to be outdone, Sun Simiao (581-682) also known as the herbal king was the first to advocate nutrition and diet for the treatment of diseases which modern day doctors like me are only beginning to see its wisdom.

The legendary Huo Tuo who was imprisoned by Cao Cao of the Three Kingdoms fame, was the first to use anaesthetics to perform surgery. Most of the knowledge of Huo Tuo died with him in prison.

I wish to zero in on one physician extraordinaire and this is Wu Tao, better known throughout the Taoist world today as Bao Sheng Da Di. This title was given by Emperor Ming Renzong of the Ming Dynasty. He has several other titles bestowed on him, like Wu Zhen Ren, Da Dao Gong, Hua Jiao Gong and En Zhu Gong. He can be known by such names and the Hokkiens in my town call him simply as Dai Tey Yar. He was born in 979 AD, during the Sung Dynasty.

He had worked as a government official, having passed the difficult Imperial Examination and was known for his kindness and righteousness. However he resigned shortly thereafter and retired to his village where he learnt and led the life of Tao. He was most famous for curing the breast cancer of the Empress Wen, in the reign of Emperor Ming Chengzu. Dai Tey Yar appeared as a Taoist priest to help the Empress. He diagnosed this by feeling her pulse from a string tied to her wrist and standing behind a screen, as she was not willing to let him examine her physically. Having successfully cured the Empress, he was given gold, silver and an important position in the Imperial Court but he declined, left the Palace and disappeared. He was then already an Avatar, where time and space he has transcended.

Many locals in Penang, where I reside, who have not been cured by modern day specialists, will seek the herbal prescription of Da Di from the temple that is dedicated to him. After praying to the heavens with joss sticks, the person will ask for the deity's help and then place the burning joss sticks across his wrist, one at a time, for the deity to diagnose. He is to shake a wooden jar that contains divination sticks until one falls out. To counter check with Da Di if this is the prescription, he must throw some kidney-shaped wooden blocks as one would throw dice, to get the answer. Once confirmed, the process of asking how many doses need to be taken is repeated by using the divination blocks. The prescription is then taken to a nearby Chinese herbal shop to be filled. There are many happy patients after seeking Da Di's help it seems.

Incredible, really, how a dedicated physician who attained the Tao in the year 1036 at age of 58 years still continues his service to many people of the world today. For sure, I have indeed referred some patients of mine to this physician extraordinaire.

I believe when you practice methods to help you go within such as meditation and when you are in touch with your Higher Self, detached from ego you will discern which guidance is appropriate for you. This leads us to the next chapter...

15. Meditation and Health

I was very surprised when some of my friends who belonged to a certain religion told me that they are not supposed to do meditation! It nearly knocked me off my chair. They were highly educated medical consultants and to me, it was a surprise that they did not seem to question anything and just followed without knowing the reasons. Others think that meditation is a waste of time while there are those who think that only gurus and eastern monks meditate.

Many people have started to meditate but have given up half way due to indiscipline, a restless mind or lack of interest when they saw or felt no benefits. There are all sorts of stories and opinions on meditation. Those who are deeply obsessed with any idea, philosophy or a religion cannot really enter into meditation as they have such a huge self-made barrier. This barrier will need to be broken down if they even want to try to think about meditation.

Let me first tell the story of my journey into meditation. Personal experiences are the best I feel as they are original. Somehow, I just knew that I needed to do meditation but didn't really have a clue how to do it. First as a very busy houseman, there was just no time to sleep soundly or eat in peace let alone do meditation. Then, there were no gurus or meditation centers that I could go to during that time. No one I knew did any meditation anyway, or for that matter pray even. Thus I left it at that but at the back of my mind I just knew it would be the right thing to do, just as I knew that Feng Shui is important in my life. In other words, I needed no proof or persuasion.

I started to buy some books on meditation but the more I read, the more confused I was. Some books were very specific and detailed but too much to do and remember and so were not useful for me. These were the Taoist books. The Buddhist books were of some help, but they tend to be very confusing and profound. I was just a beginner. Then I went for some other authors, non-religion based and although there are many good books out there, the ones I found were talking basically crap!

However, all the while, I just sat down and 'meditated', though I was not sure if the method was correct. I just remembered one Taoist who said - "Sit and do nothing" This was my mantra – sit and do nothing. Lao Tzu said "Non doing, no one is stronger than me. In not doing anything at all no one is stronger than me. Those who are strong by doing can be defeated. I can not be defeated, because my energy comes from non doing." Oh, Lao Tzu, you are exceptional. And what was Buddha doing under the bodhi tree? Not doing anything yet by just sitting he attained the ultimate! Buddha to my mind was the greatest meditator of all time.

However the level of meditation he attained is hard to emulate, or even to understand, though not impossible as he has showed it can be done. For example he would make comments such as, 'Don't meditate, be in meditation." He was saying do not be a doer, be meditation itself. He also said when a person walks, he is a 'doer', in action, but in Buddha's mind, it is just the walking, the process, and no longer a person present. In a dance, when the dance takes over, there is no more the dancer but the dance only.

I journeyed to India to see one famous dance - The Kathak. I only saw the dance, not the dancer. The performer then had attained such perfection, that he disappeared - only the dance remained. I wondered how many of the tourists saw that. I understood what Buddha meant but I still had one problem with what Buddha said about there being no God. How can an Enlightened One say such things? I knew it was not right, yet at that time the only information I had was that he said there was no God.

It was years later that I could reconcile with what he said. You see when you have a deep desire for the truth; it will be revealed to you one fine day if you really seek it. Ananda, who had followed Buddha for forty years, was as puzzled. He witnessed three different answers from Buddha in one day! In the morning, when a villager asked Buddha is there God, The Enlightened One said, 'No." In the afternoon another asked him and he said "Yes" then in the evening when one more asked him, he remained silent. The first and last answers were heavily publicized in many articles on Buddha and Buddhism until I chanced upon the second answer and Buddha's explanation to Ananda.

He explained that although it seemed like the same question, yet it was different. The first man was mentally suffering due to confusion surrounding his beliefs and so Buddha answered "No". The second man was an atheist and had seeked Buddha's confirmation. Buddha saw that this belief was causing the man much suffering and he wanted no part in causing further anguish. He answered 'Yes', so that the athiest could not say even Buddha said it is so. The last man was a much more simple and religious man, not asking for any confirmation, and although Buddha kept silent, the man went away but Buddha knew he understood what Buddha conveyed without saying anything. Then I found out that the Vedas said 'He is and He is not" and Lao Tzu said "Truth can not be said"

Doing meditation, even without any guru or solid knowledge, I was training my mind, but of course, I did not know it. I just found it to be relaxing and peaceful and also it was an excuse for me to stop doing my Tai Chi. I just had no time to do both, it was either this or that. In that phase of my life, I had a good friend who was very psychic. One night, I was supposed to meet her at her apartment but due to work, I was not able to go and just thought that I would call her to let her know. I was so busy that I forgot to make the call.

Later she phoned me to tell me what she experienced. When she got back to her place, she saw me waiting in the hall way of her apartment block and just when she wanted to say sorry for being late, I disappeared into thin air. She had seen a thought image of me as I was focused on going to her place.

She also related to me another episode of my disappearing act. Her small nephew hardly three years old, one day was looking in a certain direction in her apartment and refused to take his attention away from a particular spot - he was really staring at nothing. The family were all puzzled and started to call out to him. The little boy then answered that Uncle Yeoyeoh was there. Of course I was never near the place, but I did recall it was one of the days where I again missed the appointment to go and visit my friend as I was caught up in some hospital work. I believed this story because little kids below three are still innocent and not contaminated with the stereotyped thinking of the adult world and logic.

Whenever I go to a new place and if conducive, I sit down and meditate straight away. One day I was in Java, Indonesia and was visiting a volcanic site and felt the urge to meditate. It was such a beautiful place - it was cool, quiet and simply wonderful, being away from civilization and close to nature. During this meditation, I had broken certain barriers. I had the most immense feeling and was totally conscious of it. It was an out of this world, or rather, an out of body type of feeling. First I felt that I grew bigger in size, bigger and bigger, but I could see my physical self as the same size, then smaller and smaller as if I was seeing from a higher and higher altitude. It was such a fantastic feeling, so hard to describe – it was a feeling of happiness, freedom and one with nature all at the same time.

The message I got was I and the mountain are one; I and the sky are one, and so on. I was the sky and the mountain at the same time, by now, I was so big in size that I saw my physical body just as a small speck below. Then I got panicky and I suddenly was back down in size - as my usual self, and I came out of my meditation.

Another fantastic experience I had with meditation was when I visited one of the caves of Mulu, Sarawak (Borneo). At the mouth of the big cave, was a rock formation in the shape of a head of a giant lizard. I was amazed by the rock and thought it must be of some significance. So I just closed my eyes and did a quick meditation. Not long afterwards, I could see, in my mind's eye, a glimpse of a huge lizard, like a dragon in fact, sliding down. I knew I must have had a glimpse of the real giant lizard that had dwelled in this cave and was forever guarding it against intruders.

In another cave, this time not far from my own city, I too sat down to meditate. It was very quiet and I was surrounded by some vegetation but far away were the mountain ranges. During my meditation, I could see in my mind a huge python sliding in the forest of the far away hills just before it blended into the distant mountain.

The mind is very powerful and doing meditation will certainly improve the powers of concentration. This had been demonstrated to me several times in my own experiences. Once when I was in London, some friends took me for a short city tour and to reciprocate their kindness I told them I will buy some pizzas but when I saw the price tags, I needed to down size my own order to keep costs down. When I saw the man making the pizzas my friends ordered, I was regretting my cheaper order. I was thinking how nice if I no longer needed to be too concerned about my finances.

As my friends ate their meal, it was even more mouth watering for me. Then the man was making another similar pizza and I though he must have made someone else's order first but I was surprised when he handed it over to me. I quickly said that I did not order this type and he realized his mistake but then he said "Never mind, you take it but pay for the price of the one you ordered; I have never made a mistake in taking my customers' orders all these twenty or so years of selling my pizzas!"

So I had the expensive type but paid only for the cheaper variety. This incident left me enthralled because it was not the first time incidents like this occurred when I was thinking intensely in a certain manner.

A few weeks earlier, I was at the check out counter at the supermarket when I thought I had given the cashier a ten pound note. The cashier hesitated for a moment when she was giving me my change and added more change to give me. As there was a long queue behind me, I took the change and left. When I got back, I checked my wallet and discovered that I had given the cashier only a five pound note. It was too late and too far away to go back and return the extra money. Anyway I had a chance to redeem myself as this occurred on another two occasions unintentionally and I managed to return the extra change before leaving the supermarket. This accidental ability should not be misused.

The latest was a deliberate experiment I had performed not too long ago. I was standing outside my clinic, as I usually do to contemplate, when I saw a stray cat sitting quite close to me. I was told that we could zap bad entities with a sizzling crack of our aura when we are in the astral world while doing some astral travelling if the need arises. I decided to try and with an intense concentration, gathered my aura and formed a sharp spear to poke at the cat. Nothing happened and just when I thought it was all nonsense, the cat all of a sudden gave out a squeal, looked bewildered, and went off, not knowing what had hit it!

Still more recently, I solved a problem unintentionally by my intense concentration. I have a wall clock that chimes by the hour but the sound is too loud especially in the middle of the night and I was afraid it was disturbing my wife. So I was thinking it would be nice if the clock didn't chime at the hours eleven and twelve midnight. Many weeks later my wife brought to my notice that our wall clock did not chime at eleven or twelve anymore. She was joking about this funny clock that only chimed up till ten o'clock. I just smiled and said, "Good for you, so it will not keep you awake." However I have not yet been able to re-program the clock back to normal!

The above experiences of mine will not be the last even more occurrences have and will come, too numerous to narrate here. Some symbols I see with my Third Eye while meditating are still a mystery to me as to their meanings. I have not advanced to a great stage in meditation yet. Do not compare my experiences in meditation with your own progress there is no such thing as a better experience they are all personal and just are what they are. Everyone will experience differently and how fast or slow each one will progress, no one knows.

Those who progress very fast may do so because that they have done meditation before in their previous lives, while those who do not seem to progress at all may not have the strong desire to do so or may need to practice more. If you do not start meditating I believe your spiritual progress will be slower still when compared to others who have done some form of meditation.

Why meditate you may ask. There are also many who seem to be interested in meditation but so few are transformed by it. There are many reasons that I can think of, but suffice to say, I feel that no one will progress in the spiritual arena unless they meditate, visualise or communicate within which are all forms of meditation. All great masters and gurus meditate. If you are not interested in spiritual progress, then at least it will have a bearing on physical health. These two come together anyway. As I have said, I believe the greatest meditator must have been Gautama Buddha, who discovered so many Truths and gained Enlightenment.

Christians may say Jesus did not meditate, but I say how do you know? If certain religions or governments forbid you to meditate, then, for some it is even more enticing. There must be a reason meditation is restricted by some cultures. I think it is that you may find many truths that man-made establishments do not want you to know. When something is restricted it causes more interest - just like a story my Dad used to tell me. A boy discovered some gold in a plot of land and so as not to let anyone know there was gold, he put up a sign to say 'There is no Gold here" Sure enough every villager came to dig with their hoes.

Thus to the question why one should try meditation, the answer can be summarized as -

1. To understand the psyche and gain a more effective life
2. To create new, positive channels in the mind and eradicate those that are destructive
3. To gain relaxation and thus better health
4. To attain Self-Realization and inner peace.

When thought waves are stilled your true Self appears. It is total relaxation that prolongs anabolism and reduces catabolism in the body, so one may appear more youthful. It is a powerful tonic, with energy that permeates all cells and vibrations that can heal the body. By mastering the technique of meditation, all knowledge can be tapped into and the ego is tamed. In today's world, there are simply too many distractions. The mind and Self are being totally forgotten, remember, we are not just physical bodies. We need to be in contact with our Higher Selves.

On an every day level meditation promotes healing from within, to gain more and balance existing energy. Good health is free of energy blocks. Our powers of concentration are increased and thus we are more creative and productive in our day to day work.

The immune system benefits greatly from meditation and blood circulation is better, thus bringing in nutrition to the cells and removing waste products or toxins. There is a feeling of peace within us. Through meditation we make important contact with our souls. If your mind is without any thought, it is pure and this mindfulness can move towards the heart where the soul is. Feel the peace in the heart. When thoughts are there this can't happen. When awareness and thoughtlessness meet, it is meditation, or what Patanjali called Samadhi becoming sushupti. When you know how to relax, nothing can disturb you.

Some types of meditation are –

1. Japa Meditation
2. Hatha Yoga Meditation
3. Jnana Yoga Meditation
4. Bhakti Yoga Meditation
5. Raja Yoga Sutras
6. Taoist Meditation
7. Bhuddhist Meditation
8. Zen
9. Tibetan
10. Vigyan Bhairav Tantra
11. Others

Each of the above categories has several sub-types and can become complicated. That is why I do not follow any type per se but use my own modified method, incorporating bits of the above to what I feel suits me. All techniques are basically methods to remove yourself from the past and to allow the present to be here and now.

Hatha Yoga is famous for the awakening of the Kundalini. However I would caution those who are attracted to stimulate their Kundalini because firstly you need a bona fide guru to guide you properly and more importantly, awakening Kundalini power may not be for every one. Overwhelming feelings may result if one is not prepared or ready and the awakening is not conducted in a controlled manner. When the kundalini has united with Siva in the Sahasrara Chakra, the yogi experiences extreme bliss and attains superconsciuosness. However, very few yogis have even reached the stage of Ajna Chakra, and even those who have attained a very high level, find it difficult to control. However there are methods whereby the Kundalini is not awakened but developed and strengthened and therefore one can still be in control. One such method is the Snow Mountain method of Taoism and along with this some other preparations are required.

Some masters talk of reaching emptiness as the highest point in meditation. Buddha has a word for it - shunyata. Once you have reached this inner treasure, it will remain with you. This is the mysterious paradox - to attain deep inner emptiness, whatsoever you do or speak is not from you – because you are no more. It comes from emptiness, the deepest source of existence, the same source from which this whole existence has come. That is why Hindus say the Vedas are not written by man but the divine – God Himself had spoken.

There are some dangers in meditation that I feel must be told as well. Some will reach quite a high level and think they have attained the highest and best level and become stuck in the astral world by the illusions that may trap them there and in fact impede their progress. Many such "gurus" have indeed fallen into this trap.

They were really in other realms that were not beneficial to their spiritual progress. The way to deal with this is not to be attracted to the fantastic illusions that will entrap you. Just note this "paradise' and move on. Always have your own belief steadfast – be it Lord Buddha or Jesus, and entities of the astral world will leave you alone.

The other danger is to meet entities that say they are so and so (God, Buddha, Jesus and so on) and lead you astray with their kind of preaching. Always test them and do not just accept what ever they say so easily.

In Vigyan Bhairav Tantra, there are 112 methods of meditation to suit many individuals. These methods are for people of past, present and future. These techniques were narrated by Shiva, more than 5,000 years ago to go beyond consciousness. In Tantra, everything is divine, thus there is no such thing as the devil. If you read the 112 sutras given by Shiva, you may not understand the instructions.

For Tantric meditation, one needs a guru to explain in depth what the sutras intend you to do. In the first sutra - Shiva said "Radiant one, this experience may dawn between two breaths. Focus on nothing after breathing in and just before the next breath comes – the Beneficence."

Buddha used this method and he attained Enlightenment. Since then it was known as a Buddhist method with the name Anapanasati yoga. The trick is to watch the gap between the two breaths that is all. This is always the paradox. So simple and yet so profound. Many spiritual masters have used a method of the Tantric meditation with their own modifications.

Gurdjieff learned a technique in Tibet from Buddhist masters who actually taught him Sutra 25 – "Just as you have the impulse to do something, stop". Krishnamurti had once said "No need of meditation, don't meditate." He was just like one of my feng shui masters, who had never meditated. He had very deep knowledge but was quite an arrogant guy and one day I asked him, "But sifu, have you ever tried meditation?" He said that was one thing he never experimented with and thus he could not continue any more conversation with me on this topic as he had no experience. I had managed to hurt his ego and the next time we met he knew not to put on any airs with me.

So, as Swami Sivananda said, "No more words, enough discussion and heated debates! Retire into a room, close your eyes, have deep silent meditation. Destroy the imagination, thoughts, whims and fancies; withdraw the wandering mind and fix it on the Supreme."

Below is a basic method of meditation:

1. Regularity of time, place and practice are the most important factors for successful meditation
2. The most effective times are dawn and dusk, when the atmosphere is charged with special Spiritual forces. The preferred time is between 4 and 6 am
3. Try to have a separate room for meditation. As meditations are repeated the powerful vibrations set up will be lodged in the room.
4. Face North or East with spine erect. It is not necessary to place the legs in the classic lotus position. Any cross-legged comfortable posture will do.

5. Before beginning, command the mind to be quiet, forget the past, present and future.
6. Begin with 5 minutes of regular breathing and then slow it down.
7. Keep the breathing rhythmic. If a Mantra is used, coordinate it with the breathing.
8. Do not force the mind to be still, this causes disturbing brain waves. Simply disassociate from thinking and just watch it.
9. Select a focal point for the mind to rest upon - for example the dantian or third eye. Never change this point.
10. Focus on a deity or up-lifting image, OM may be used.
11. Begin with twenty minutes and later progress to one hour and never more.
12. Do not lock the room; make sure the phone will not jolt you when it rings.
13. If possible, slowly phase out meat and intoxicants - a vegetarian diet is best.
14. Expect nothing and you gain more. Expect something and you gain nothing.
15. Do not be happy when you gain special powers, it will lead to your downfall.
16. Never think you have gained Samadhi, for it is just an illusion.
17. If you really want to progress, you will need a Guru.

"When the student is ready, the Guru will appear"

Never be afraid if you meet Astral forms for they can not harm you.

For most of us, meditation is not for spiritual advancement but more for inner peace and relaxation with added health benefits. I strongly recommend that all should try to meditate and not bother what benefits it will bring, for surely as the sun rises, the gifts will be there, though one will not know in what aspects they will be. I am hoping that medical schools will look into meditation as part of the curriculum of medical students.

Before this chapter is concluded, I wish to teach another simple but very effective technique of meditation that will protect you from attacks of the spiritual realm. Forever have in your mind's eye, that you radiate pure light from your entire body. Hold this image always. Hold it when you walk, talk, work; all the time when you are conscious. Radiate light and love. You can imagine or visualise or think of the light in any way, it can follow the contours of your physical body or just be a ball of spherical light radiating from your body. May the Force be with you.

16. The Ultimate in Preventive Medicine

Before giving my ideas of the ultimate in preventive medicine, let me discuss the antenatal classes that are conducted in most hospitals. This may sound like a sweeping statement but I think they are of no use! From what I have observed, although the contents of such classes vary from centre to centre essentially they are similar.

Most are dealing with details of labor, the possible complications of pregnancy and giving birth and how the heroic doctors can solve them. There is usually a lecture on pain management while in delivery and some topics on baby care. Post natal exercises are also taught. These basic topics are covered by all antenatal classes and I think it scares the parents more than helps them, especially when they talk of the complications. Some doctors conduct these classes to enhance their egos by giving very technical talks, forgetting that these are not medical students.

Many of my patients ask me why I do not conduct such antenatal classes for them and I tell them that my classes will be conducted during labor itself! I also add that whatever was taught before labor will all be forgotten and so it will be a waste of time. During labor and at the second stage, I will teach them how best to avoid unnecessary pain, when and how to push etc.

Good antenatal care goes a long way towards a safer pregnancy and birth, there is no doubt. However, this will not guarantee that the baby will grow up to be emotionally and psychologically stable. The world today witnesses a lot of crime, wars and social unrest, and each day it is getting worse. Yet no one knows what to do to stop what some believe as a slide to hellish conditions on earth!

Actually the ancient Chinese knew more about mother and fetal bonding than our Obstetricians of today. They knew the importance of such imprinting on the fetus that will have an important bearing on the psyche of the baby. These have since been known as superstitions by modern folks and so the younger generation pay no attention to them.

Such knowledge was seen about 3,000 years ago in ancient China in the Zhou Dynasty (1100 – 771BC) where mothers to be are advised to see no evil, hear no discordant sounds and to speak no words of annoyance during the entire pregnancy. (It was also recorded during the Qin Dynasty (221-206 BC), Western Han Dynasty (206-24 AD) and advocated by Xu Zhicai (550-577) and the famous Tang Dynasty physician, Sun Simao (618-907). The best recorded history being that of Tai Ren, the mother of Zhou Wenwang who later became King Wen of Zhou)

Students of I Ching will be familiar with King Wen who had contributed to the I Ching, The Book Of Changes and to a very accurate method of divination using the I Ching via a calculation he devised. This method of calculation, called the King Wen method is not easy to muster and it took me two or more years to decipher the steps and yet I can only be 90% accurate. I always say that if my answers are inaccurate, it is because of the mistakes I make in the calculations and not the I Ching itself.

Tai Ren had taken all measures to make sure her unborn child had the best of external and internal conditions to nurture his growth in her womb. When this child grew up to become King Wen, his wife in turn practiced the same method his mother did and his son, Zhou

Wuwang, later became King Wu who was able to completely over throw the Shang Dynasty (600 – 1100 BC).

When I was living in London, a friend of mine had mentioned that her son told her that while in her womb, he used to know when she opened her mouth to eat food as he could sense this action and had a memory of this. I was quite sceptical when she told me this until I had an opportunity to ask the son who was then a tall ten year old kid. He maintained the same story of how he could remember, while still in his mother's womb, he even shared that whenever his mother swallowed some food he felt excited!

My mother, NGK, also told me that while she was pregnant with me, she grew a craving for mangoes and there was a huge mango tree near our small house. She would stare at the ripe mangoes and wish that a mango would fall so that she could eat it. One fine day a mango fell indeed! Now I am very fond of mangoes and remembered vaguely this incident but I could not place the time sequence of how and when I could remember this story!

When mom told me this, I was confused and stated that it must have happened after she had given birth as I somehow remembered it, yet she insisted it was before I was born! When I heard the story my friend in London told me, I recalled the day my mom told me her story of the mangoes, I knew mom was not wrong, it had actually happened before my birth and yet I recalled this episode. This truth is mine to keep.

Another of my recollections was very puzzling to me for years until I discovered the truth behind it. When I was below three years old, my father showed me a mirror and I got the shock of my life when I saw my reflection! I was completely traumatised and cried incessantly for hours; being so shocked at my 'face' which I remembered did not look like that. It took several days to calm me down after some Taoist prayers were done by Dad. When I was about five, I used to run to the mirror to see my face and was so puzzled at why I looked like this, an Oriental, as I thought I was completely different in my look, more Middle Eastern.

It took a long time to accept my Chinese appearance and then I grew out of this obsession to check my face in the mirror by the time I went to primary school. The explanation is that I remembered the face of my previous life and thus it was a great shock to see my face in this life, which is a total contrast. This was my first experience of reincarnation, I have several others but I am straying off topic!

What I want to convey in this chapter is that scientists are still unaware of how much a fetus in the womb can have cognizance of his external environment and can thus be positively or negatively affected. This to me is a crucial factor in bringing up ones children. Helping them start with a solid positive foundation makes all the difference in which direction their lives will proceed.

Fetal memory can be explained by the esoteric view point, which to many scientists, can be regarded as bordering madness but I will still share this knowledge! The soul does not reside fully in the developing fetus but hovers around the mother. Perhaps about one sixth of the soul may reside in the unborn to guide in its development. The time where the soul resides fully in the body is debatable even among the masters of esoteric knowledge.

It is believed by some that during the first breath of the new born baby is where the soul enters the body fully. Others are of the opinion that it isn't until around six to twelve years old. Thus the developing fetus is not so innocent and devoid of feelings or consciousness. Since this is the case, it is vital that the family must not quarrel, fight or curse, especially the pregnant woman as these negative emotions will have an imprint on the fetus. If the atmosphere surrounding the family is detrimental in terms of feelings and emotions, the fetus absorbs these negative traits and a similar kind of intellect and behavior ensues.

It is little wonder that so many wars have been fought in human history and are still happening. The fetus being imbibed with emotions of fear, anger, hatred and jealousy in utero and then after being born, these negative energies are still in his surroundings, re-enforcing what has been picked up in the womb.

So you can see why I do not conduct antenatal classes like the others, it really serves no purpose. However to conduct classes on how to have positive imprinting to the unborn is a different matter - I may then contribute to a society that will be more forgiving, loving and co-operative. Actually this will be my coming project!

Recently I came across the great work done by Dr Zhi Gang Sha and I was greatly surprised that we share almost the same ideas, especially with regards to karma and also about the theory of suffering by humans through disease and life. His contributions to the knowledge of soul advancement is beyond any doubt the most practical, easily attainable, important and far reaching advice than anything I have known or studied. It was very strange, that his book answered all my prayers and confirmed what I knew my self.

In my daily meditation, I had set aside some time to ask God that I may have access to Wisdom and Knowledge. I also experimented with the dream master so that in my sleep, I let my soul go and learn something important in the great libraries of the Universe. However I lack the power of recall and so was no better off when I woke up in the morning.

Sometimes, even when not meditating but in a semi-meditative mode, I talked to my soul, saying what a shame that you, my soul, with so much knowledge, experience and wisdom gained through the ages in countless rebirths, are unable to tell me things so that I will be on the right path and waste no more time with wrong decisions. It was not long after this that I discovered Dr Zhi Gang Sha's work and am now following the spiritual exercises he recommends.

For the first time, I actually heard the voice of my real Self, my Eternal Soul. I recommend that all those who are serious in improving themselves seek out his books.

It is so interesting, right at the same time, I also received material that was so well written about there being no such thing as soul; reincarnation and that all the reports on having come back from death are utter rubbish. I just smiled at the test that I felt was given to me. This is Yin and Yang in action. Sometimes it is just pointless and a waste of time and energy trying to convince someone to believe what you believe. I always say to these people that they have all the time in the world to discover their own truth. Take your time and all the knowledge that you require to find truth will be presented to you.

This brings me to conclude this topic. I believe the ultimate in preventative 'medicine' is to have a peaceful, conducive environment for a pregnant mother to carry her baby, in addition to making sure she has a well balanced diet and healthy lifestyle.

Ideally, as suggested by master Ivanhov, the pregnant mother is advised to be isolated in a special resort, away from the negative vibrations of city life for the entire length of her pregnancy. This heavy investment is worth every cent because the newborn would have been protected antenataly with good nutrition, soothing music and relaxation of the mother via meditative techniques. It is an atmosphere where anger, worry, and other negative emotions are reduced as much as possible as are the harmful effects of modern appliances like TV and mobile phones or nearby high tension cables.

Children born in such manner should grow up as useful, healthy, peace loving and gentle citizens. When more and more such children are brought into this world, we can expect a better world where peace, love and a feeling of brother and sisterhood prevail. These children will be useful and productive citizens.

Crime rates should naturally fall. All categories of crimes such as burglary, serial killers, hate crimes and crimes of violence can be traced back to traumatic childhood experiences. I also believe that many negative imprints started while in utero. This perhaps explains why being born into a household environment where the fathers are drunk, violent and the neighbourhood is infested with crime, homeless people and junkies can lead children into such a lifestyle. Negative exposure that starts in the womb and continues throughout their childhood and teenage years is a hard habit to break.

It thus seems that no matter what sociologists and psychologists do, crime of all sorts keeps escalating because many children are raised in these environments. Not all men and women are born equal this is the sad truth of life. It really depends on where you are born and subsequently how you are brought up. Where you will be born in your next life and to which family is the million dollar question!

However even being born can to a certain extent be 'controlled', like the Tibetan lamas have done. It is sheer supreme mind control developed by years of meditation. For ordinary people like us, we can try another method that requires life long awareness, of right living and conduct in the hope of enjoying a happy life and therefore a better rebirth.

17. The Age of the Internet.

The world has changed tremendously, wondrously at times and at others not for the better. I often think that wow, we are in the 21st century, am I so lucky. However this bubble of euphoria has burst several times. I realized that there is great progress as well as great regress.

The sayings by our seniors of those good old days sometimes really hold true. I had mentioned earlier about LaoTzu, who was so disillusioned with life in ancient China that he sat on his water buffalo and went up the mountains never to be seen again. That was almost 2,500 years ago! I think things have not changed one bit from the view point of Lao Tzu – the greed, crime, corruption and warped thinking of humans. The only thing is that it is in a bigger, more sophisticated and atrocious scale than during his time.

I feel it would be a good thing for all of us every now and then to pack our bags and head for the peace and quiet of somewhere like the Himalayas to recharge our batteries! It is beneficial in this internet age to just take off and go out in the wilderness in order to come back to our lives refreshed and able to look at things from a higher and more serene perspective! We can use this time free from the media, the constant pull of the net and all outer distractions to reflect within or study and ponder the laws of the Universe.

Upon my studies I discovered that the ancient Hindu sages were also right on target about the good old days. Their Golden Age (Satya Yuga) lasted for 1,728,000 years and all were just perfect.

Then followed the Silver Age (Treta Yuga) which lasted for 1,296,000 years and where evil and corruption begin to show up.

The Bronze Age (Dvapara Yuga) ensued where disharmony, evil and corruption gained a strong foot hold.

Finally we end with the Iron Age (Kali Yuga), which will last for 432,000 years and where evil, greed, famines, diseases, wars and corruption are at their height. We are now at the Age of Kali Yuga. Time in the Hindu concept is like an inverted vortex. You may have felt yourself that time and manifested thoughts seem a lot faster as one travels down the vortex which is explained when comparing the number of years for each of the Ages.

This is also in agreement with the Buddhist/Taoist concept where karma is now getting faster to manifest, perhaps in the same life time of the person.

The Yugas are comparable to the type of civilization achieved during the time of Atlantis. Of course many will protest to say Atlantis did not exist and there are no archeological records of its civilization. For many students of esoteric science, Atlantis was real and the level of its civilization was far more advanced than where we are today. Their scientific advances made ours look like kindergarten.

Now I understand better why even in this modern time, our progress in some areas does not even match what had been achieved thousands of years ago by some long forgotten civilizations. The moral decay is now so evident, younger and younger people are getting pregnant and the increasing numbers of incest cases are being surfaced. In other words, the good old days of our grandparents were really the good old days.

Patients nowadays are also a different breed altogether, unlike patients of yesteryear. In this day and age people demand more in every respect which is not a bad thing but sometimes it is just counter productive. I think even doctors who are sick should leave the management of their condition to the doctors who are caring for them.

Many patients will now surf the net for medical information or they stumble upon a site where they find what they think they are looking for. The problem arises when they choose to believe all that is written on the net rather than the expertise of their real life doctor. This can lead to fear of the complications of treatment or their disease when it does not apply in their cases.

However it is an uphill task to re-educate such patients who think the doctors are not revealing the whole truth or that these doctors know nothing of their disease or conditions. Many lay men do not know that by reading one article on the internet, newspaper or Sunday magazine, a doctor they are not. In fact, no matter how much they read, without well informed guidance one is never in a position to make the wisest of decisions

I am surprised that many patients think that just because something is on the internet makes it absolute truth and their reading of it can lead them to important decisions based solely on this information. I usually do not spend my time or energy once a patient shows that he has a very strong opinion because of reading an article or articles that have not been written by specialists in the field. I would only say that I am always here to be of service if they need me in the future.

This type of approach will shock them because they really enjoy showing off what they have read. Secondly, they expect you as a doctor to defend your stand strongly, but to me if it is not a matter of life or death, I leave you to be what you want. There are patients who will come to see you but tell you what medication to give them. There are many more case scenarios of patients making your job difficult or even interesting, if you look at it in a humorous way.

As I have emphasised in an earlier chapter, we shouldn't always blame the patients when doctors can be difficult to deal with too, whatever the reasons. It never ceases to amaze me at the kind of medicine that is given by some doctors or the methodology used in the management and how some of our local pharmacists play doctor.

Personally I feel it is best not to read about your condition if your intention is only to challenge the medical diagnosis. However, if you want to know more about your medical condition and you can not get enough input from your doctors, then I feel reading about the ailment is justified, to satisfy your curiosity.

Leave the choice of drugs and drug combinations to your experienced doctor. Honestly, I would not recommend you to spend your time reading medical articles, rather I would say you spend that energy in a more beneficial way which is to meditate and visualize you are getting better and that your doctor is doing everything correctly.

There are so many websites that sell pharmaceutical drugs, herbals, Ayurvedic and Chinese herbal medication these days. It is hard to gauge the quality, safety and authenticity of their products. Remember the medications available from these sites are to be consumed into your own body and I believe whatever you consume (food, drugs or drinks) must be safe beyond doubt.

Fake drugs are a real danger to one's body and many are indeed available through the internet. Not only can the body suffer from purchasing dubious drugs from the internet but there is an avenue here to find anything you are searching for not just information and products but also people who bring mental and emotional stimulation.

Many marriages are broken because of one spouse being involved in a clandestine relationship which originated from surfing the web. I bet the number one past time in some very strict, sheltered or religious families, where there is much restriction, is surfing the pornographic sites and chat rooms.

Gamblers can play games or place their bets on-line and gamers can play video games till the cows come home. Sweet talking con artists prowl the singles websites in search for their victims. Not too long ago, the mobile phone alone was responsible for so many changes in our lifestyles and now it is the internet.

There are addicts being formed – some have to check their emails or social networking sites often. Then there are download freaks – they keep down loading material just in case they need it or some other excuses are being used to justify their actions. Information over load can be reached easily.

The virtual world has indeed caught up with the real world. Viruses can infect man or machines now. Thus you have viruses, Trojan horses, worms, malware and spyware that can knock out your computer. Lucky for humans, they are not physical infections! The issue nevertheless is how the virtual dimension can still affect us. This is scary as we will be more and more dependant on computers in our daily lives and computers of today, I predict, will be replaced with even more powerful models that will make today's latest version look archaic.

I have spoken only of the negative side but of course, for every degree of negativity there is the opposite degree of 'positivity', this is yin-yang balance. The internet has completely changed many lives in a miraculous way. It has brought the world to our finger tips. We can communicate with people all over the planet in a way we never have before. The good old days of snail mail and waiting three weeks for your letters to come from overseas has been replaced with instant mail! Not only that, we can now talk and see our friends who live overseas just as if they were in our own living rooms by installing a program on the PC and all for free!

People have been reunited with long lost loved ones and families by joining social networks. Anything we need we can just look up on the internet, from songs, translations, dictionaries, spell checkers, maps, books, pictures of absolutely anything, hobbies, encyclopaedias, you name it the internet has it!

We can even book hotels, plane tickets, seminars without picking up a phone, a wallet or moving an inch from our computers. It truly is a marvellous invention and just like us needs to be taken care of by making sure we feed it well. Computers have many a time been compared with our minds and so we must install information which is compatible and delete all unnecessary programs to avoid dis-ease or virus infection.

18. Coma, Dreams and Sleep

This topic is included because I feel it needs to be understood by all and especially the relatives and friends of those in a coma. I am not saying that doctors are exempted from the subject but it may be hard for a majority of them to accept what is being written here.

There are several causes of coma and we are not here to discuss the medical aspects, rather what it really means in the esoteric sense.

Basically a patient in a coma may have all body functions working but there is no consciousness or there could be some other organ damaged, usually the brain after some trauma, surgery or disease. There are many cases whereby after several months or years, they will awaken and regain their consciousness. Thus it is a very difficult position to come to a decision of whether to continue the medical care or pull the plug, so to speak.

The way I think about coma cases is that they are in a way an indirect proof of the soul principle. The body and brain are there, but comatose with no responses of a living person. Then sometimes, for no apparent medical reason, the person wakes up, albeit having some deficiencies of some kind occasionally. Their personality may even be slightly different from before the coma due to residual medical causes or they could be like a totally different person altogether, in which case medical personnel will be unable to give a logical explanation.

The esoteric viewpoint is that the soul left the body, which is now only a shell with no consciousness. It is about the soul going somewhere to contemplate his life – to decide whether to continue with this life and this family or to call it quits and move on to other experiences. That is why it is being encouraged that the family members continue talking to them, updating them on current events of the family and surroundings, assuring them of the family's well being because they can hear for sure. Communicating with them may help to ease fears they have of returning.

Their soul usually will be hovering around their body off and on. When they finally make up their mind, either they come back into the body to regain consciousness or they choose a different path and move on in their evolution and their body will shut down and die.

I will relate to you the fantastic story of a close cousin of mine, let's call him Heng. Before I begin let me give you a little background before the miracle. Heng in his childhood was among the most mischievous kids in the village. He was chased by his mother, my aunt, all over the house with a cane most of the time. He was also the most hilarious practical joker of all his siblings, who were almost as naughty and mischievous as Heng.

I remember my auntie used to yell at the top of her voice all the time when we visited their atap house. He was several years my senior and so I was spared of his practical jokes.

Any way the years rolled on, Heng married a very young girl who was still at school and he was then working as a Customs Officer, his final occupation. Even in his adulthood, he would pull practical jokes on many of us. Making us laugh was his specialty – by his ways or his jokes. I always looked forward to meeting him whenever I was in town.

As he aged, he had several medical ailments and complications, perhaps from his lifestyle of sleeping late, boozing and cigarettes. By then I was a medical doctor working in the government service and being transferred here and there. When ever we happened to meet, he would ask for my medical advice or opinion, not that he took the advice at all. He was rather proud of the medical problems that besieged his stout body and enjoyed making fun of doctors and nurses. We never had a dull moment when we met.

He was under the care of this consultant and that professor from the University Hospital and was admitted every so often to stabilize his several problems – hyperthyroidism, hypertension, diabetes, hyperlipidaemia, renal insufficiency and cardiac problems from angina, fibrillation to heart attacks. Amazingly he was ever so cheerful and the whole ward would roar with laughter and before long the whole hospital got to know him.

Finally he was forced to retire from service because of his poor health and this also affected his income and they were getting poorer and poorer until most of the furniture in the house was sold off and we would have to sit on the cold hard floor when we visited him at home. Most of the time, unfortunately, I would meet him in the hospital ward, well at least I'd have a decent chair to sit on.

He also picked up some medical jargon and was very proud of it, being able to discuss medical issues with me like a real professional. Not bad for a guy who hated studying in school and played truant so often.

One day I got a call from his wife who said he died in hospital. This is what we all feared and it happened. The consolation was that the consultants were puzzled that he hadn't passed on years earlier. His case notes were made into volume one, two and etcetera and it gave me a headache just to skim through the piles of notes whenever I saw him in hospital.

So Heng had finally departed for the happy hunting ground. I made my way to the hospital and was going to the mortuary where his body was kept. I remembered he even made a joke of this - he told his wife she must know how to get to the morgue as one day she will definitely have to go there to claim his body and as for me, since I am a doctor, I will know the way. The heck I know the way – the hospital is so big I lost my way most of the time.

On my way there, I received another phone call on my mobile advising me not to go to the mortuary - they found he was still alive and in the intensive care unit! What? It seemed even in death he was still playing his practical jokes? If so, I said to myself, he'll be in big trouble, for the entire clan had been informed! I was getting a bit frustrated, having almost reached the morgue and then having to find my way to the intensive care unit, another maze to go through both in the hospital and in my mind. This guy was something else. Was he really alive? He certainly would have a lot of explaining to do when I meet him, I thought.

Sadly I found him in a serious condition in the ICU and comatose. I remembered being a busy government doctor; I could not stay or wait in hopes he might wake up. I however got recent updates from the family and finally heard he was discharged and resting at home!

As it happened, I still could not meet up with him for some years after the episode due to my busy schedule and being posted again to an area some distance away. Slowly news trickled in via our other relatives and his youngest brother. It seemed that Heng had completely recovered from all his medical ailments, almost no trace of them! He need not take any medication where he used to have a mountain of tablets of every color, shape and size. This was the second miracle; the first was coming back from the dead!

He was certified dead by one of the senior consultants who had even signed the death certificate but later when in the morgue, someone noticed him breathing again and quickly called the emergency team who was able to resuscitate him. The senior consultant who signed his death certificate was red faced and the joke of the hospital.

Now the third miracle was that he gained some special powers to predict events in the life of people and became very good at locating missing persons. He got to be very famous and started to get ang pows (money in red packets) as his rewards and his house was filling up with brand new furniture and even a TV.

I was determined to meet up with him, no matter how busy I was. So very late one night I arrived at his house and we met again. He looked the same old Heng but hardly joked and was rather more serious. He showed me a Dragon Chair that some happy client had presented to him for solving some kind of problem.

The Dragon Chair must have cost thousands of dollars and all I know is that such chairs are for no ordinary person. In Chinese culture, it is reserved for the Gods. Any way we had a lot of catching up to do.

He told me that since his discharge from the hospital, he had been very religious, reading Buddhist and Taoist books and saying prayers of all kinds. One day, he had a message in his head, saying that a man will ask him something and he will know the answer and from then on his life will be different. He was puzzled.

Indeed, one fine day a stranger knocked on his door to ask for some directions. He inquired whether Heng knew the whereabouts of a certain person. This person was not contactable and had been missing for a long time. Heng was surprised that he blurted out the location of the missing person.

The stranger it seemed followed Heng's directions and located the individual and so word got out that Heng had an uncanny power. Since that day, streams of people continued to flock to his house, asking for the whereabouts of loved ones and all were found with the information Heng gave. He told me he didn't know how he knew the answers.

His reputation grew enormously and he was being rewarded by red packets of money, as is the tradition among the Chinese for services rendered. From being below the poverty line, he became quite comfortable and able to replenish his previously bare house with furniture, TV set and so on. We then adjourned to have supper of herbal pork soup to celebrate his coming back from the dead. I visited him quite often after that as it happened I had more free time and we would talk late into the night.

I learned that he was being employed by a karaoke lounge owner to bring in business because whenever Heng was there, more and more customers would just appear. Heng was being paid quite handsomely plus free booze and food as long as he showed up and he would go every night. So it was back to his old lifestyle of late nights and being hopelessly drunk.

His latest clients were mostly the underworld gangs, since his information was valuable to these gangs who were tracking down ex-gang members who had double crossed them. Families with runaways came to see him less and they dwindled to very few.

In one of my visits to Heng, he told me he was helping a lady who was in great financial difficulties and was running away from the loan sharks who were harassing her. Loan sharks in our place are well known for their no holds barred tactics to extricate money with huge interest from any clients who have defaulted on their repayments of the loans taken.

It was the suggestion of that lady to go to the Casino and try her luck to win some money with Heng's help to pay off her debts or her very life would be in danger when the loan sharks came next. Reluctantly, Heng was sort of forced to go along with the idea and off they went to the casino and lo and behold, she managed to win quite a good sum of money that night. Heng thought he had got rid of her but she came back several times to pester him to take her to the casino again and again.

I was at Heng's house on the particular night he was to take her to the casino for the last time. We had some idle talk and he was getting ready while waiting for the lady to pick him up. I left Heng's house as it was quite late and I had a long drive back to my place, some 20 or more kilometers away.

That was the last time I saw my cousin Heng. It seemed that they went to the pub and karaoke first before going to the casino and while drinking his beer, Heng had a massive heart attack, fell from the stool and died with his dancing shoes on, so to speak. This time it was for real and he could not be resuscitated. Again the entire clan came to bid him farewell.

He was the talk of the family and town. He was given a second chance to live and thus in repayment for this new life, I believe he was to perform some meritorious acts along the way. That was the reason he was given a special gift. However, the wrong kind of people came to ask for his help and he got himself involved indirectly with underworld characters. God had to take back the special powers bestowed upon him.

I wish to relate another story told to me by a high ranking Police Officer several years ago. This Police Officer had a course mate, Mansor, who was also his room mate and both were under going training to be police cadets several years ago.

The officer noticed that Mansor was an odd person, preferring to be alone all the time and seemed to be talking to himself or to someone imaginary. Although Mansor was never good in his studies, he managed to pass the internal examinations with ease. Being his room mate, my friend asked him about his odd behavior. Mansor decided to spill the beans.

Mansor was told that as a child, his parents said he was very religious and pious. One day he fell into a nearby river and was drowned. They were preparing him for burial when someone noticed that he moved and they got him to hospital to be examined further. He slowly regained normal health after awakening from the coma he had slipped into. As the months went by, his parents noticed that he was not the same as before, he was more mischievous, naughty and hyperactive. His parents accepted this new behavior of his and would always mention that the old Mansor was really no more. He had no recollection of his childhood at all.

While undergoing police training he used to get visits from a very beautiful girl whom only he could see but no one else and that was why it seemed like he was talking to himself. He fell in love with this beautiful girl. It was she who would tell him what topics to study to pass the exams which he did with flying colors, while class assignments were always done so badly.

The girl of his wakeful dreams even took him to visit her relatives, again who were visible only to him. Years went by and Mansor married a real lady but he was still visited by his first love in the nights. His real wife had accepted this strange behavior of Mansor.

Rising from the dead is thus not that rare and does occur. If I had heard from others, I would think it as just rubbish, but the case of Heng my cousin which I encountered first hand and the serious Police Chief's narration had given me some valuable information on the unknown.

In the case of Mansor, it is known as soul migration, with a new soul inhabiting the body of Mansor and the coma was a period of adjustment for the new soul. In the case of Heng, the soul was the same, as his memory was intact and he recognized all of us in the clan, his friends and others. In both situations, death was documented and funeral arrangements were made. I am sure there must be hundreds of equally bizarre stories such as these that go unreported.

In a similar vein to coma cases, the condition of Alzheimer's is getting more attention. Doctors are still trying their best to cure the condition. To those who are unfamiliar with this condition, a brief medical description is given here. The onset is insidious and subtle, with early memory being affected. There is lack of initiative, irritability, forgetfulness and loss of concentration and thinking faculties. Then there can be a change in mood, mainly apathy. There can be easy fluctuation from laughter to tears. Paranoid ideas and delusions can develop. Depression and anxiety can manifest also. In the late stages, extrapyramidal signs appear and they walk in short shuffling steps. Finally they may lose the faculties of speech and movement as well as thinking ability. There can be marked increase in confusion with possible lapses into coma. The best example the world knows was that of Ronald Reagan in his last years of life.

The esoteric interpretation of Alzheimer's disease is as follows. Some souls are undecided when they ought to leave the body and they take an experiment, so to speak. They leave the body for short periods of time to explore the other spirit worlds and come back to their bodies again. This explains the short memory loss and irrational behavior and then full recovery. Later, with more courage, they leave for longer periods of time and so the physical body is like a shell again, with no response to external stimuli. Finally, when the soul has made the final decision to permanently leave the body and earth, the afflicted person dies. Thus I ask you, how can drugs cure this disease?

In cases of sudden death, the opposite happens. Let me explain. In sudden death like those that occur in motor vehicular accidents, the souls usually are unaware that they have died. This creates a special problem to the soul concerned; they are caught in a world which is neither here nor there and become hungry ghosts according to Taoist belief. Although rituals are performed to guide the souls to their rightful abode, many still refuse to go and so they stay around the earth plane, especially at the site of the tragedy. The same applies to suicide cases. I shall relate these two types of scenarios with some incidences.

My good friend of my early years in Kuala Lumpur city told me this. His nephew, who was in his teens, had died in an accident while riding a bike. After the funeral and 100 days later, family members could sense his presence. They then consulted a Taoist medium. The medium revealed that actually the dead person was in turmoil because he did not realize that he was already deceased. He was puzzled and troubled why family members were not responding to his interactions at all. The family had to conduct special prayers again to send the spirit off.

In other cases, those who finally realized they are dead feel a lot of anger and frustration because they think their lives were snuffed out before their time. They too become stuck in this dimension and suffer the realities.

My own relative told me this about her father-in-law who committed suicide more than twenty years before she got married into the family. Her husband's family had wanted to sell off their flat but found it was almost impossible because potential buyers would suddenly back off from their offers and transactions would not occur at the last moment.

The family consulted a medium who told them that their father's soul was still present and resented them for selling the flat and was the cause of the sudden failures in the deals made. They were shocked because his suicide by jumping off the balcony of the flat was more than twenty years earlier. They believed the explanation because at times, family members thought they had a glimpse of him occasionally but each did not believe in what they saw nor brought the subject up. Again special prayers were required to send the soul to its rightful place and not long after that, they managed to get a buyer.

The science of sleep and its companion - dreams, are still being studied in sleep laboratories and I can say that not much is known for it seems the scientists are day dreaming. The science lab is really not the place to study these topics. The gurus or Taoist priests that meditate perhaps are in a better position to deal with the subject.

Sleep is just like a coma; for we lose our consciousness, we don't know where we are. Some people say they never dream. The only person I know that stopped dreaming was Gautama Buddha, for once attaining Enlightenment; there is no need for dreams. Since we have not yet attained anywhere near arahatship we must still dream in our sleep but many of us don't remember.

During sleep, the body works very hard to recover, recuperate and regenerate. For children, it is a time of growth. That is why children need plenty of sleep. Sleep deprivation in the most extreme but highly rare cases can result in madness and even death, as reported of young, healthy adults that die from playing internet games for long periods at a stretch.

Those who meditate deeply will find that they do not require much sleep. In fact, as one of my very early former gurus had said he was awakened by the Gods very early in the morning when he felt too lazy to wake up for meditation. Later he discovered that he really did not require that much sleep anymore when he meditated deeply and regularly.

He told me this because I gave the excuse that I have no time to do meditation and he suggested for me to wake up early to do so before going to work, however I countered with the reason that I needed lots of sleep and he came up with this story of the gods kicking him out of bed at an unearthly hour to do meditation.

In the early hours of the morning just before we wake up, our blood pressure goes up and this is a medical fact, which doctors attribute leading to a higher incidence of heart attacks seen in early hours of dawn. However I have another explanation. When we sleep, our souls are so happy to be freed of the confines of the body and they travel to the astral planes and at times somewhere on this planet itself. The early hours of the morning is when the soul comes back and the body is startled and therefore blood pressure rises for a short time.

We interpret or remember this as a dream. This is an important mechanism to maintain good health and a sane mind. Imagine if you are confined to a small cage all your life, it is just unbearable. The soul feels this way with the body. This to me is the main reason why we need to sleep and the dreams that occur are those episodes we remember in our brain when our soul is out of our body.

To those of you who are more aware and spend time on consciousness development, you may experience 'real time' when you dream. Here you are aware that this is not a dream. The things you perceive in that sort of dream are real. I have had such experiences on several occasions, sometimes on consecutive nights.

One of the most weird experiences was that I would fall into space, but keep turning in a vortex, seeing stars, the dark night sky, sometimes worlds all turning in a great circle and speed, and then a "normal' dream will ensue. This happened every now and then for many nights in a row and I would be aware of the phenomena starting again, yet powerless to stop it.

The sensation of falling and going round in a circle in the darkness is not a really good feeling. It is like being sucked into the eye of a hurricane. At times, I remember I only flew in a straight line, hurtling through the dark skies and seeing stars far away but zooming past many of them at a great speed.

At other times, our dreams are a recollection of events from a past life. So if you remember your dream, you could have a little insight to what important events had occurred in a previous life to warrant such a memory of it. Are dreams real? Well, I had a dream that left me speechless.

I dreamt that I was walking through an arched gateway and into a white building. There was a huge pool, like an Olympic pool. It was shimmering in light, nearly blinding my eyes. There were women in traditional Indian attire pouring water at the four corners of the pool. Many months later, I asked a friend to take me to any Sikh temple in town. I just had the urge to visit one for no apparent reason I could think of. I was not familiar with the town as I had recently been posted there.

This lazy friend of mine kept delaying until one day I cornered him and he had no choice but to make a definite appointment. He promised to take me to the biggest Sikh temple in the town. On the way there he changed his mind and decided to take me to another

Sikh temple even further away from the town. I said any temple, just as long as we went to one.

It was a long journey and finally we arrived at the temple. As I got out of the car and walked towards the temple I stopped dead in my tracks. I was shocked at what I saw; it was unbelievable. In fact I had to lean against the car to catch my breath. My friend was not aware and he just went straight to the temple grounds.

I was so shocked because every detail of my dream was right in front of me - the archway at the gate, the path leading to the temple, the temple itself - all were just as I saw in my dream, with only one exception - there was no swimming pool. As I wandered around the temple, still in a daze, I know why there was a swimming pool in my dream - it was the very shiny marble floor. It was so shiny that it looked like a pool with very still water when seen at some distance and at the right angle!

After doing some prayers and a quick meditation at the temple, we left. I was still catching my breath. This could only mean that I was really there during my dream. Unless you have had such an experience, you will not understand how I felt – so confused, it was even a little disturbing as my scientific mind could not explain, and no one could interpret the meaning of my dream.

A close friend of mine knew of my unusual experiences in life and especially of my nightly dreams and when ever I visited he would poke fun at me by asking 'Where will you be flying to tonight?"

These days I make use of my sleep time to improve myself. I have already mastered the art of waking myself up at the times that I intend and it is always right on the dot. No need for alarm clocks. Now is to perfect the art of giving myself specific instructions for soul advancement during my sleep. Yes, we can still make use of sleep to further advance our knowledge!

19. Big and Expensive is better...

I had been working in the government service for many years and my prolonged stay was due to a few reasons, among which was that with the public hospitals run by the government, my expertise and knowledge could be used for the poorer section of the population as those better off usually go to the private hospitals.

In many places in the world, private hospitals or clinics are associated with better service and a more comfortable setting. The waiting time too may be less than in public funded hospitals run by the government. If one was to work in the private sector, especially in larger hospitals, we have the security of knowing that our patients would obviously be those who can afford our services.

Since I had come from humble beginnings and had not forgotten it was the government clinics and hospitals that my parents could afford to take us to when we were ill, I had always shunned away from those large private hospitals and preferred to remain in government service to give back to society. My idea of being a doctor is to treat as many people as possible and not just a select few.

Like so many others before me, I was later very disillusioned with government service and resigned to join some private enterprises. My experience in the private sector was not that ideal either and I finally worked independently. I have thus tasted life in both sectors which are really like two different worlds.

Today, the health industry has evolved in many ways and grown even more complicated. The management now may interfere with the doctor's view point on patient management issues as money is involved. It is worse still if the management is headed by non–medical personnel who do not understand why certain methods of patient management need to be conducted.

Things get even worse when insurance claims are involved and other third parties like private health management organizations get into the picture. A simple case of patient management is now complicated with so many intervening and interested parties. The patient may thus get exploited; the doctors get frustrated with management issues and orders that come from above. Thus gone are the good old days of patient care. Yet this is seen as progress.

The cost of health care keeps going up in almost all countries and it is the poor that always suffer. Although inflation and other acceptable explanations will increase health care costs, many other reasons are artificially created and thus unacceptable. The monster keeps growing more powerful and if nothing is done to revamp health care issues, the collapse of the health industry will surely occur. The bubble must burst once a critical size or situation is reached.

Years ago, we could still use some very effective drugs or antibiotics that are cheaply produced for specified conditions but now some of these drugs and antibiotics have been discontinued. I discovered that the disappearance of these useful medications are not due to problems of drug resistance exhibited by the clever disease causing agents; but rather to the introduction of better and more powerful alternatives which of course are much more expensive. Subsequently some drugs which were available loose, in large quantities have been discontinued and are now all dispensed in blister packs, again making the costs go up for the patients. The reason given was that blister packages, where each tablet is safely encased in a bubble on a plastic or aluminium strip are safer in terms of storage and transportation.

There is a common perception amongst our local populace here that the bigger and more expensive the hospital the better. They think they will get superior and more powerful medications and the doctors are better skilled to save their lives. It is of no significant financial consequence if rich people patronize these hospitals but it is a disaster when poorer patients believe in the same concept.

I have seen, heard and known many cases of poor patients selling their houses or borrowing money from friends, relatives and illegal loan sharks just to pay for their medical bills. Yet many times, in almost all cases of terminal cancer, they will die and their immediate families are left with a big burden and debt, making matters much worse than before. It is really tragic if you have seen it with your own eyes how these surviving families go down the spiral of no return. And all because every one subscribed to the idea that the more expensive the hospital and doctor, the better the outcome.

Of course there are several more reasons for less well off patients to shun public hospitals but whatever their reasons are, I believe they are not justified. There are some rather smart folks who are choosing to be treated at government hospitals even though they can afford private health care, like a few of my friends. They believe that they should not spend so much money to the extent of depriving their loved ones the funds needed for their education or their living expenses as the public hospitals here in Malaysia these days are at par, if not better than the private hospitals. My message here is to inform that for all chronic illnesses, cancers or otherwise, and all cases of emergencies, it is often better to get to our public hospitals. Most public hospitals locally have been upgraded and their facilities can be at times just as good as the private hospitals.

Emergencies whatever these may be are best sent straight to public hospitals, do not even waste time getting to private clinics. This statement is applicable almost 95 % of the time. It may really save the life of your loved one. Clinics firstly are not well equipped to deal with emergencies and other factors like lack of well trained staff and medico-legal implications make them quite unwilling to accept such cases and thus precious time is wasted in the clinic itself.

Private hospitals will accept emergency cases but some of them do request a substantial sum of money to be deposited before further action can be taken and this is a waste of time if the relatives have to raise that amount of cash on the spot. Thus, in my opinion, real emergencies should be sent to public hospitals at once, mainly to save precious seconds and later so as not to burden the patient or their families as the costs involved in public hospitals are much more affordable.

I wish to comment on house calls now that we have dealt with where to go in case of emergencies. I believe almost no doctors today will do any type of house calls and the reasons I will discuss perhaps are applicable to this part of the world where I practice. The most important reason these days are that it could be quite dangerous for a doctor to answer a house call as he may be robbed or even kidnapped!

The contents within the medical bag he carries will probably not be able to contribute much to the management of the patient, thus it is again a waste of precious time. It is better for the family to get the person to a hospital or call for an ambulance if they have no transport of their own. I have done a few house calls and that was only because I knew the family well and the kind of ailment the patient suffered from.

Even so, I would discourage them to get me to their house; instead I would ask them to bring the patient to my clinic where everything I require is at hand and if impossible to do so, to call for an ambulance straight away.

There is another issue to discuss for the benefit of the public. Many who have medical insurance will find out that they were not covered for certain procedures and it is too late when an emergency is at hand. It is important to know what one is entitled to so as to be sure of admission rights and not be caught unawares.

There are also people who want to be admitted on the most flimsy excuse just because they have medical insurance coverage and have not used the facility. I find it shocking! I have even heard about how parents wanted their kids to be admitted even though they can be treated as an out-patient simply because their medical insurance is under utilized! In over crowded hospitals, this is taking a bed from someone who may really need it.

In the panel clinic system as practiced here, there are again many who do not know how to think for themselves. I have had several patients who are under the panel clinic of their company and since their insurance does not include blood investigations, they would rather forego this vital step in their management than pay for it themselves. Thus the monitoring or diagnosis of their condition is hampered.

They should not jeopardize their own health in this manner. This way of thinking is widespread among panel clinic patients; it some how becomes a consciousness that they shouldn't have any medical treatment unless it is free and they will not pay from their own pockets. I feel rather frustrated that I am not able to contribute more effective care and in fact these patients would think we are always trying to get them to pay out their own money to boost up our earnings. This is sad.

The other extreme is the patients who will walk into any privately run laboratories to do all sorts of blood tests on their own, believing that it is cheaper and sad to say, many of them have been taken for a ride. The attractive laboratory test packages are advertised as very cheap where in actual fact, my patients are shocked to know that I can do better and more tests for them at a much more reasonable cost. To add insult to injury inflicted, these laboratories sometimes have inaccurate results as in false positives and false negatives, they are not doctors therefore they are unable to interpret the results as accurately and often just hand over the reports without a word. Some even have the guts to interpret just to sell some dubious products to correct their test results.

Many layman do not know that these tests can not rule out a medical problem entirely, that is to say, to have a normal result does not mean that their health is excellent, for there are many cases whereby despite a normal result a few weeks earlier the patient still ended up with a fatal heart attack or stroke.

On the other hand, a healthy looking person who undergoes a routine wellness health check, ends up being diagnosed with a serious disease and is subjected to even more tests which can be invasive. If this proves to be true, then the effort could have saved his life. The question then is to look for a caring and competent doctor that has access to an accurate and reliable laboratory. Health care is not a DIY thing.

There is now the emphasis here in Malaysia on medical tourism. This will bring lots of revenue for the government and the private hospitals concerned. The idea is very good - those whose hospitals back home are too expensive can fly here for a holiday and get some medical issues sorted out as well. The only losers will be the poor, as usual. The hospitals and doctors will then be interested to cater for these richer foreign patients, thus pushing the costs of medical care up. The poor will then be the neglected lot and treatment is getting more and more expensive and I believe it is only time until our public service hospitals will need to put their prices up anyway. Then the poor will really be suffering.

In view of the above facts discussed, it then boils down to keeping ourselves as healthy as possible. Good health is indeed most important and valuable. It is always the case when one loses something that is taken for granted only does one realizes its importance and sometimes it is just too late. For many families, if the husband is the sole bread winner, then he is the most important link in the welfare of the family and thus his health is of utmost importance. Many men fail to understand this and they are among the worst culprits as far as taking their own health is concerned.

Too often many folks depend on the health care system as the only way to solve their health problems. I too have emphasised this throughout the book that we must consult our doctor for health advice. We always tend to look at the external world for most things like material happiness and fulfilment. It seems much easier to go to a friend when we have concerns or spend time on social networks such as Facebook on the internet and so on.

I also have said life is about yin-yang balance – for every outside activity we need to balance it with an inside one. We tend to forget to look within on a daily basis and some aren't even aware that our bodies and minds have incredible powers to overcome most emotional and physical ailments by themselves if we just know how to communicate with our organs and cells; if we learn how to listen to them. Dr Zhi Gang Sha has even taught how to do a soul order to heal ourselves for his theory is to heal the soul and the body will be healed, which is what I have always believed.

20. Time to be a Vegetarian

I used to gobble up my food due to my hectic schedules as a doctor. Worse still, I ate just about anything and was still able to maintain my weight without doing much exercise. One day, due to some circumstances, I decided to become a vegetarian for a year. Although my weight still did not change, I felt so much lighter and alert. It was then that my other senses grew sharper.

When I was initiated to a certain Taoist temple as a disciple of a Taoist master, I took the vow to be a vegetarian but only two days every month. I even go into a semi-fasting state when I am unable to find vegetarian food for the two special days. Meditation, fasting and being a vegetarian is just a natural process for many on the spiritual path. Just like mixing with bad company, committing crimes, doing drugs and things illegal is natural for those playing a different role in this drama of life.

To non- vegetarians, it is inconceivable not to have animal proteins in the diet. They will say they will have no more strength, although like so many people, they only lead a sedentary life style! Many other excuses only a non-vegetarian can think of will be put forward by them, some of which I can't even conjure up in my mind.

On the other hand, I have come across even toddlers who will spit out any meat given to them, even if it is blended into baby food and they often grow up to be completely vegetarian, some becoming monks or nuns in their life. These souls are special ones not that anyone who becomes a vegetarian will be a monk or nun.

Vegetarians are more likely to be less aggressive, less hot tempered and more compassionate people. They are less likely to have cancers but this is not the rule, since cancers are completely something else as we discussed at length in an earlier chapter. Medical theories on the causes of cancers are only academic, not the whole truth.

Some vegetarians will not eat certain products of the plant kingdom like onions. It is often those on religious diets like gurus, monks, yoga instructors etc who think that these are aphrodisiacs and not to be taken. Some vegetarians I know profess to be religious but can commit all the crimes a crook can think of!

I can say this because I had a personal experience with a full time vegetarian who goes to temples and even speaks of what Buddha preached yet she was so full of poison in her mind and heart it was unbelievable. So there you are - the drama of life and we chose what we want to be.

Buddhists, Hindus and some Taoists like me do not consume beef, the Moslems shun pork, some believers of Kuan Yin avoid a certain type of fish, I took a vow of not eating dog meat as well, not that I had ever eaten dog meat!!(In this life I mean). The Chinese mad monk, Ji Gong relished dog meat yet he attained the Tao. Buddha ate whatever he was given. I don't know of any religion that forbade its followers to eat vegetables. If anyone does, please call my hotline!!

My Dad fed me beef soup when I was small, he took me to the stall under the trees for this special dish and bought beef home to cook as well as I was crazy over beef cooked with spices and pepper. However when I grew up, I had a natural disliking for it and avoided it altogether.

One day in London, my friends took me to Chinatown for some food. After just a mouthful, I could not keep it down. I did not realize it was beef and my friends did not know I don't eat beef. The whole day I felt uneasy.

I had a friend who worked part time in the horse racing stables, to clean and feed the race horses. He said one day they had eaten some horsemeat when one horse was destroyed after suffering from injuries. The next day when he returned to work in the stables, he noticed one by one the horses were uncomfortable with his presence and one horse even kicked him, this never happened before he ate horse meat! Yes, I truly believe in my heart it is time to be a vegetarian.

The livestock industry is responsible for 18% of all anthropogenic greenhouse gas emission. In 2008, a country like Brazil lost 12,000sqkm of rain forest to cattle ranchers and soy producers for European animal feed. This is a pity, to clear the forest to grow crops for animal feed instead of agriculture to feed humans. Livestock rearing can use two hundred percent more water to produce one kg meat than in growing wheat.

Kilogram for kilogram, beef and pork can produce thirty times more carbon dioxide than other protein rich food like beans. Methane gas can heat up the atmosphere by as much as seventy two times more than carbon dioxide while nitrous oxide is more than three hundred times more potent than carbon dioxide.

Ammonia gas is the main cause of acid rain and ecosystem acidification. The largest source of methane, nitrous oxide and ammonia is from the animal industries. Moreover, hydrogen sulfide, a pollutant from the animal industry depletes oxygen further. The animal wastes and chemical fertilizers to grow soy and corn contaminate our water supply and can reduce the ocean's oxygen and kill marine life.

As a comparison, it takes 23 gallons of water to produce a pound of lettuce, 25 gallons of water to produce a pound of wheat, 49 gallons of water to make a pound of apples while 815 gallons to produce a pound of chicken, 1,630 gallons for a pound of pork and 5,214 gallons for a pound of beef! The water resources for human use and consumption are being depleted and wars in the future will be to secure this life giving water, not oil.

Now it seems that one ounce of processed meat per day increases the risk of cancer of the stomach by 15% to 38%, while for colorectal cancer the risk is by 21%. For vegetarian men and women an early death risk is reduced by 50% and 30% respectively. This gives food for thought really.

A Harvard study of more than 40,000 healthy professionals showed that those who ate hot dogs, salami, bacon, or sausages two to four times per week increased their risk of diabetes by 35%. While those who ate these products five or more times per week experienced a 50% increased risk.

Anatomically our digestive system is designed more for a mixed fruit and vegetarian diet, as seen from the types of teeth we posses and the length of our intestines. An occasional meat diet will supplement whatever vital ingredients our body requires. Even in the days when animal meat was not contaminated with artificial hormones, antibiotics and beta agonists, the very act of slaughtering animals will pour out emotions of pain, fear and panic in them, and as I have stated in an early chapter these energies generated were and still imbibed by people who eat these meats.

In more modern facilities, the methods of slaughtering are less traumatic but I believe animals have a sense that they are meeting their end anyway and these emotions are still generated nevertheless.

On the human side, those who work in such places are responsible for inflicting so much pain and anguish to these animals and they really have blood on their hands. Karma created will need to be repaid in one way or another, in a time near or far off, in this life or in the next reincarnation.

Though one may argue they are only earning a living to feed themselves and their family, but then we do have a choice to change our method of livelihood. Another reason to become a vegetarian.

Perhaps one may go step by step, experimenting with a diet more in fruit and vegetables and reducing the amount of meat, substituting animal protein with that from fish. Life first emerged from the sea, and food from the sea is again more suitable for us than land animals.

The food chain concept is very important. For meat eaters and non-vegetarians, the chain is like this – sunlight to plant, to herbivores, to carnivores, and to man who eats meat. In other words the cows, elephants and horses eat the vegetation whose energy comes from the sun; it is already second hand energy! This is still good as can be seen by their strength.

We, who are eating beef and so on, are getting energy third hand, which is now less in value. Of course if we can ever absorb sunlight energy directly, it would be the best. In fact, a few Eastern mystics who have managed to do just that do exist.

One Indian holy man was thoroughly investigated by doctors under strict scientific protocol and he was documented not to have eaten or taken in any water for the entire length of the observations. This man claimed that all he ever needed was to look at the sun. His alimentary canal had shrunk extensively due to long periods of not using it and from not eating anything for years, an indirect proof of his claims. This in fact is the highest yoga methodology – the yoga of the sun.

In the engineering world, scientists are working on cars that run without petrol as this commodity will be exhausted in the future and to reduce pollution from such engines. First are the hybrid cars that run on petrol and electricity. Even in the world of cars, the petrol is being discarded for more energy efficient power generation with fewer pollutants (vegetarianism).

Since oil is actually a source of pollutant, some believe it is why Mother Earth had locked this from the face of the earth. However, clever humans dig deep oil wells to release it to the surface and use it as a form of energy, by releasing pollutants to the air from its combustion.

Another esoteric teaching about why we have venomous animals and reptiles is that the amount of poisonous thought forms created by humans feed the production of these poisonous reptiles that inhabit the Earth. Yes, it's time to be a vegetarian!

Far into the future, if it happens that carnivorous animals start to eat vegetation, despite the abundance of prey, it means that finally Earth will be in for a long period of peace and love. The loving thoughts and actions of humans will gravitate down to the animal kingdom as well. As above, so below.

21. Time to Discard Negative Attitudes

It is my observation that many people have negative attitudes and thinking. This can be seen in daily life everywhere. The attitudes include selfishness, rudeness, hatred, jealousy, envy, racism and the practice of black arts. In Malaysia, as in many other countries as well, bad driving attitudes, road bullying and selfishness have contributed to many road accidents and mishaps resulting in loss of time, money, suffering, disabilities and needless loss of lives.

Traffic jams here are mainly caused by inconsiderate and selfish drivers parking haphazardly, jumping queues and not giving way to others who have the right of way. They occupy the centre of a dual carriage way, not allowing anyone to overtake while driving slowly.

Some who are about to leave their space in a busy parking lot despite spotting that you are waiting for them to drive off deliberately prolong moving for as long as possible. This is either due to complete inconsideration or simply just to irritate you! This has happened to me on several occasions but I just wait patiently to park, sometimes even losing the parking place to some one who is so uncivilized as to rush in to park before I can do so. As a result, everyone suffers just because of a few bad drivers.

The way to deal with this constant and daily harassment is to adopt an attitude of peacefulness within. Before driving off somewhere, do some mind work – imagine your drive is smooth with no traffic hassles. When you experience a lovely time driving on the road, acknowledge this, feel happy and remember it. One other trick I use is to tell myself that I am not here to teach these rude and inconsiderate drivers a lesson, let others do the job. Then I feel better and the incident does not spoil my day.

Poor unprofessional road building and planning are also factors that have contributed to many accidents. There was a toll plaza along the highway in Malaysia that had so many terrible accidents with loss of lives that the authorities had to demolish it and move it away to another location and reduce the incline of the approach.

However many of us who knew the area, the reasons stated are in addition to poor sub-standard designs by incompetent engineers; the land was the burial ground of the local Orang Asli tribe, the indigenous people of the land. We have to respect their ancestral burial ground. In Australia, Ayer's Rock is a must see tourist attraction but sad to say many tourists seem not to honor the sacred place and there have been cases where people who took some rock samples home as souvenirs suffered immense bad luck.

Getting rid of selfishness and inconsideration leads you to more treasures; the world has enough opportunity and riches for everyone. I wonder have you ever stopped to think how fortunate you are to be born a human?

As a matter of fact, I was told that there is a very long line of eager souls who are ready to incarnate. They just hover round their parents waiting for the correct moment to enter the womb. Should the parents decide to abort the pregnancy, then they have lost a great opportunity to be reborn and will have to wait again for a long period for the correct time. What if you were an animal, or a plant or lowly bacteria.

As far as Buddhist teachings go, it was never on record that a human fell from grace and had to be relegated to be reborn as an animal. It may be thought that all humans have undergone aeons of transmigration from an evolving cell to plant and then animal existence and finally graduating to be born as a human. You may have come across animals that were outstanding in their lives; say for instance they saved their human masters from death in a fire or from drowning.

It is my belief that such animals are the likely candidates for 'uplift' in their soul evolution to be born as a person. However in their first lives as a human they would need to learn a lot, thus some people with animalistic attitudes and some genetically deficient syndrome babies with low mental faculties could be the manifestations of such.

I do not think it is possible for an animal consciousness to be reborn as a musical talent in their next birth as a human. Likewise a maths or musical genius would be a consciousness that had retained their abilities built over several lifetimes and are able to remember and express their skill in the present life.

Many people take their lives for granted, wasting the wonderful opportunities to improve themselves and to evolve to a higher level in thinking, acting, behaving and so on. They squander their precious human lives doing things that are negative like taking drugs, robbing and plundering others or even to the extent of killing another human being, sometimes using the name of God.

If only they had taken a golden path, using their physical state in this world of matter to purify themselves and to contribute something back to society or mother Earth. However, sad to say, the majority of people in all walks of life create more problems for themselves and their loved ones rather than helping to solve their issues.

Life after life, incarnation after incarnation, they repeat the same mistakes. They can't seem to break free from the chains of karma. Their karmic debts keep accumulating all the while.

I am not asking everyone to save the planet but it is the little things that mean much more like being considerate, polite, helpful, patient, respecting others, understanding people, doing meditation, a forgiving attitude and taking care of ones parents and so on. It just makes sense to do positive things even if you do not believe in the karmic angle.

In many Asian countries today, it is appalling to know that children are abandoning their parents in hospitals and old folks homes. Some even abandon their families or children. It was amazing that Confucius could see this happening and thus had a strict code of ethics to instil in the fabric of society in old China.

Perhaps Singapore is the only country in the world that has a law to prosecute those who abandon their aged parents to correct the alarming rate of such acts. The rising cost of medical care, cost of living, inflation, bad attitudes of the parents themselves towards their kids or their own parents are all factors that in one way or another have contributed to this present state of affairs.

Among the negative emotions that is very common and that have caused serious damage to relationships, divorces, hate crimes and so on is anger. There is so much anger these days. Not only is anger socially destructive, in Chinese medicine, it hurts the liver. Hate causes rage in the heart, worry eats away at the spleen, sadness depresses the lungs and fear afflicts the kidneys. These negative emotions will eventually cause damage to the respective organs and ill health results. Consequently it affects both the internal and external worlds, to the delight of the dark forces, which feed on such energy.

To overcome negative emotions from taking a hold on us, one must learn to meditate on peacefulness and happiness. You may concentrate on your breathing, aware that you are breathing in and then breathe out. Be conscious of this unconscious act. Make sure they are deep breaths. In this way, you will get the blessing of Babaji, an avatar.

If a person's thinking is negative or one is stressed, worried or doubtful and the third Eye is open, he or she may see many entities with a similar energy vibration in places like gambling dens, prostitute houses, bars where lewd behavior predominates and other places of ill repute.

The best way to deal with such negativity is not to suppress it for sure one fine day, with all the suppression, it will simply explode. Buddha had a very effective method, which I have only now realized how much wisdom is behind his method.

He recommends you just be an observer - observe your anger arising, observe it going away, all the while saying and doing nothing. Just observe. In this way, you do not suppress it with force but just let the energy dissipate by itself. This method is the best way to dissolve the energy called anger. To those who understand deeper, Buddha had even advocated to observe a man walking, but really to see walking as a process but not the man. Indeed anger has caused many a misery – families are broken, marriages spoilt and friends turn into enemies. I think if one is able to control and dispel this energy, many will gain so much and hearts will not be broken. I urge you to look into your anger and deal with it.

Crime rates are on the increase everywhere, in almost every country. People involved in crimes like murder, rape, incest, robbery and other heinous acts are in the younger and younger age group. Building more jails, stiffer sentencing by the courts and more law enforcement units are not the real answer.

One must address the root cause which I believe lies in the incessant battle between good and evil. Dark forces strive on negative feelings of fear, hatred, jealousy, envy, anger, ego and lust. When many people project negative and black thoughts, these become thought forms, a kind of energy that will be attracted to similar receptive individuals and they are then influenced by these negative energy forms. The cycle amplifies as more and more people think negative thoughts.

Such behavior, if not checked, can affect an entire population of a nation and so bring destruction. I believe there are such things as the Dark forces and these came into existence aeons ago. They were more interested in negative energies while the others were more into spiritual evolution and advancements. Love is the most powerful energy that can combat the dark. Mystics have always said God is Love and Love is God. Just imagine, if suddenly everyone in every country has the feeling of love towards humanity, all wars would stop suddenly as well as acts of terrorism.

I don't believe the negative thoughts of someone will just disappear after his death, on the contrary, one will not just be wise or suddenly enlightened but I think they will carry on the negative ideas, illusions and thinking to affect their lives in the astral and mental planes.

Most of the messages coming from mediums may not be those from Masters but from disembodied spirits that are full of illusions and some maybe from misdirected devotees, priests, rabbis, swamis, politicians dressing in astral forms of Masters and delivering their misguided messages through these channels.

I am being reminded of a case handled by a mystic from somewhere in Greece. A girl was being possessed by spirits and was brought to the mystic to be exorcised. It seemed that the girl was overcome by a husband and wife spirit that had belonged to a couple who had so much hatred for a certain type of race that they continued their evil ways in their spirit forms. They refused to believe that they had died so their spirit was trapped in the astral world for them to continue their hatred. You can only pity these misguided and trapped souls.

That is why Buddha taught us that we must be in control of our minds with the right words, thoughts and deeds. Right thinking goes a long way to purify ourselves. If we form a good habit of thinking of the pure land of the buddhas, along with benevolent thoughts for all sentient beings, at the time when death approaches, then these pure thoughts will be part of our vibration and this will help our departing consciousness to journey where pure, wholesome thinking resides.

This in a nutshell, is the Buddhist vipassana meditative technique. The soul will not be trapped in the warped thoughts of hatred and racism.

The ultimate plan of death and destruction brought about by terrorism and a nuclear war precipitated by the actions of dark forces serves only one purpose – to stop souls from having a vehicle to reincarnate and thus a chance to re-invent a good life of light and love, retarding the progress of life on Earth which in turn will affect the entire solar system. We must not fall into this trap. It is vital to have peace and harmony on earth as elsewhere. It is time to discard negativity.

Here then is an opportunity for each individual to contribute to world peace and harmony by focusing on positive thinking. Collectively, if each and every one of us does the same, the force unleashed is unimaginable. So here is the explanation to those that say how can just an unknown and insignificant person contribute to the world's welfare. Now that you know it is possible you will also know that each person can make a difference.

Since every thing is but energy, and energy can not be destroyed, it can only be transformed, like water into steam; we have a chance to transform negative energy into positive energy. Sometimes we face the greatest test, a negative episode in our life. So how are we to make use of this opportunity to convert it into something positive?

There are two methods, depending on the situation. In one, we just accept the lesson given to our soul. It had to happen, as nothing happens by chance. And notice that I wrote 'our soul' and not to 'our body.' All spiritual lessons are meant for the soul's advancement. If one has been robbed, it has happened. Just accept it and move on, rather than holding a grudge in your heart towards the perpetrator. In fact you could forgive the person because for him to rob you, he must be in a worse situation. Any way, the robber had created negative karmic energy for himself while you, for some previous reason, have paid back and so no more owing to the universe.

Another method may be applied by the mind. Suppose you had a bad quarrel with a friend. You can play an image in your mind of the incident, but with a good and happy ending like you are good friends again. In this way, you have a better feeling within you and also you may be surprised that your friend may take the first step to make up with you.

Actually I use this method quite often. When I see an accident on the road, and have no opportunity or time to render help, I will play back the incident in my mind but with a happy ending – for example: that I helped the accident victim to hospital.

So let us all turn negativity into positivity. It is a perfect chance to advance our souls. Those on the spiritual path may wonder how come they suffer even more when they take this path, the answer may be that you are being given more chance to clear your backlog of karma.

22. We Are All One

In the previous chapters I have touched on health and its esoteric implications and also of subjects that may be of interest to health conscious people. Most of what was written involves the individual but now let us expand our consciousness one more level up.

In many Eastern teachings, it is emphasized that in reality we are all one. Chinese mythology states that humans have existed since the earthly Mother received Qi. Her two children, Fuxi and Nuwa, married each other and had common ancestors. Nuwa established the first law in China to abandon the practice of marriage between siblings. Fuxi went on to devise the practices of worship, the Eight Trigrams, and taught how to fish and hunt. Funny, most of the world has only heard of Adam and Eve. As strange as it must feel to hear it, we are all brothers and sisters. This simple statement is now being realized by the scientific community with the genetic data that is available and still being analyzed.

Physicists realized that matter is made of atoms and atoms are made of electrons and many other sub-units. Between each sub-atomic particle is space. And when you go even deeper, even these particles disappear and there are only wave-forms of energy. Eastern mystics go even one step beyond - behind energy is only consciousness. It is a shame that we have wasted at least three or more thousand years of knowledge to appreciate only some aspects of ancient wisdom.

In the private world of theoretical physics, the Quantum Theory is really a description of probabilities and physicists know that something you do here is linked to something happening there, regardless of distance. This is described by complicated mathematics. For Einstein's General Theory of Relativity, in simple words, it means matter here causes space to warp there which causes matter over there to move and in so doing, causes space over there to warp.

The case history that I am going to relate will show how real this is – that we are all one. It was noted by many that there is a rise in childhood asthma in Trinidad of late, a trend seen in many countries too. Researches have linked this phenomenon to the sand and dust being swept over by strong winds that blow across Africa and that head towards the Caribbean as the number of asthmatic cases that needed hospitalization coincided with the sandstorm in the African continent.

Somehow the sand contained the fungus of the Aspergillus species and this also affected the coral in the seas of the region with a disease that was not seen before. The dwindling coral life then affected the natural habitat of the marine life that depended on the coral and so diminishing the fish population. The catch of the fishermen thus dwindled and affected the local food source. This chain of events spanned across thousands of miles and all life was affected.

In another case, caribou herds are dwindling in numbers across North America and it is suspected that this chain of events was triggered by a small rise in temperature of the region due to global warming. The temperature rise was just too fast for the animals to make adaptive changes. The warmer and longer summer months were ideal for insects like the mosquitoes to breed and the swarms pose a huge problem to the herd, biting them and feeding on the blood.

It was observed that the vegetation was lush due to the warmer weather but the caribous preferred to graze at higher altitudes where the climate is colder and where mosquitoes are absent. The much harsher conditions expended more energy for the herd and also the vegetation was scarcer as opposed to the lower lands with lush vegetation.

Then the higher temperatures resulted in heavier snowfall during winter as more moisture is available. This made escaping from predatory wolves much harder and more were falling prey to wolves. The decline in caribou threatens the livelihood of the native people there which for thousands of years have depended on caribou meat and fats.

Malaysia blames the hazy conditions that result in dangerous quality of the air on the burning in Indonesian plantations and small holders while Indonesia blames it on Malaysian companies that invested in plantations and this issue repeats year after year.

At the time of writing, Indonesia is having their election and their politicians have a field day in bashing Malaysia to divert attention away from the more pressing issues of economy and the eradication of poverty.

If we look into the political situation of many countries, we may be able to gauge how the morality of the country measures up, apart from getting information like the corruption index of countries. The in depth knowledge of a political situation of a country requires one to actually live there for a number of years while the corruption index is a very quick guide to gauge the situation. I have to comment upon politicians because if you were to observe carefully, they are perfect case examples if you want to study human greed, selfishness, sacrifice, ego, racism, fanaticism and sometimes intelligence.

Self–interest to amass power that leads to wealth is the bottom line for most politicians these days. They may bleed the country dry. The great heroes of yesteryear are indeed hard to find – people like Mahatma Gandhi comes to our minds easily. For a more recent example, Lee Kuan Yew of Singapore, who almost single handedly contributed so much for his country's development, although the younger generation seems to have forgotten the struggles of their grandfathers in building up the small nation.

At the time of writing this book, The WHO had just officially declared a pandemic of Influenza A type H1N1 in the midst of the worst economic downturn in decades and where many countries are yet to recover. These few examples suffice to let us know that we are all one and what happens in one corner of the world will eventually affect the rest. This is the esoteric message and yet how many of our scientists and politicians are aware of what Mother Earth is trying to tell us?

According to many sources, the world will go into upheaval and chaos will reign. This shift in energies and the earth's polarity will bring about natural disasters like floods, fire, earthquakes, volcanic activities, pandemics, tsunami, famine, drought, hurricanes and typhoons that are of greater intensities than ever experienced before. Of course many lives will be lost apart from destruction of infrastructures, economies and untold miseries. At the same time, human factors like crime, lawlessness, terrorism, genocide and political upheavals will erupt. In these times, which could have already started or the foundations are being laid now, man will understand that we are all one when they learn to help one another and that something which has occurred in another part of the world will affect them directly or indirectly.

Those who still think in terms of race and religion only will one day understand that this line of thinking is not for the greater good of the whole. It seems time and tide waits for no man, these people may somehow find themselves removed so that the whole may be freed of resistance to their evolution and progress. In other words, the world will be cleansed of people who don't understand the light and choose to remain in darkness and their souls may be hibernated until such time when they are called back, perhaps when a new world order is being created again. That the worlds or even Universes will come to an end is not hearsay, for what can be created, may also be destroyed.

What has a beginning will have an ending. This cycle goes on and on, in the micro as well as in the macro world; or as above, so below.

It is an esoteric law that anything that divides belongs to the dark forces and anything that unites, belongs to Love and Light and enlightenment. Most believe it is the final destiny of our soul to unite with the Divine Light eventually.

It recently occurred to me that the symbol of division in mathematics – a dot above and below separated by a dividing line, signifies the separation of heaven above from earth below.

Some believe that there may come a time when heaven no longer has anything to do with earth, withdrawing its blessings and that chaos will reign. However, if one believes in polarity then the light can never go away or leave but it can appear to when you are unable to see it. In order to see the light we must be open to the possibility and focus upon it by being positive and loving.

Negative ideologies, policies and politics that divide a nation will never attract light for they signify darkness. It is never too late to focus on all things positive and in so doing help the Earth to evolve towards a bright future.

The world is now divided into nations but I envisage in the distant future, countries will unite, like North and South Korea as well as China and Taiwan. Then national borders of other countries will vanish, as the nations of the world unite as one. First, this must start with individuals before families, local communities and then whole populations of nations and between nations can be united. It always starts with one, then two, then four and then many, as in the Tao.

Do not wait for another person to change for the better, start with yourself. Every journey begins with the first step, your step. As you become a living example, others will follow. The Tao will flow. It is amazing how selfish some people can be by only thinking of short term benefits for their own selves, but that is all they will attract, while those who think of long term benefits for self and others will receive them.

Some people have learned the concept of the now but are applying it in a negative, self defeating way. Let me give you an example. My cousin's husband died of a brain tumor and his mother started to ransack my cousin's house for money and valuables left behind. The old lady managed to clean out the house of many valuables whenever she visited her daughter-in-law. This resulted in a very estranged relationship between my cousin and her in-laws. She is left with almost nothing and has to earn a living now for herself and a young son. The in-laws had no regards for the welfare and future of their own grandson at all with such behavior. It is unbelievable, yet such a common occurrence. Of course every thing happens for a reason, so they say.

I ask you to reflect upon what your views are on life? If you say that you are happy not wanting to harm anyone but just leading your own life minding your own business, then I feel this may not be quite enough. If individuals are stagnant and not passionate about their own life, the lives of others and the Universe then what is the point of them being here! I often wonder if people understand the value of being a human. I feel it is a very unique privilege to be given a chance to transcend ourselves and improve our spiritual standing in the Akashic Records.

The key is to contribute, help and serve all others, with no ulterior motives for self gain. This is perhaps the single most important line in the entire book. Many people read lots of books but only a very few will try to practice the new found knowledge themselves. Millions of people pray daily, but almost everyone prays for themselves only, or for their immediate family, at the most.

I strongly believe and suggest we pray for the peaceful transition of Mother Earth. There are many who speak of our earth herself being in turmoil with climate change occurring. The possibility of the polar ice caps melting away due to a rise in world temperature will be disastrous for life everywhere. This shift in temperature is mostly man made. Our activities are destroying our own habitats and it is a simple ecological fact that if the habitat is destroyed, you will destroy the inhabitants.

How can we think positively and see the world in a better light?

You are what you believe. If nothing is being done to improve our thinking, habits and behavior, then imagine the scenario in the future of basic necessities like food and water resources becoming scarce. Wars will then be fought to have control of water resources and land. Food will be stolen instead of money as an every day crime as money becomes worthless when inflation is at an unbelievable level. Is this what we want to create?

In the above paragraph, I mentioned Mother Earth. If we still think in terms of race, religion and country, as some governments are advocating, we are very narrow minded because we are denying the fact that there are others on our planet and to think selflessly is to think of other humans as ourselves.

Our lives are really going global and borderless. In fact I consider myself a universal man and am trying to think in terms of the universe and cosmos in order to further expand my consciousness. For those who wish to understand in a logical orderly way perhaps it is time to gather what the scientists and physicists think of the universe and it is best to begin with its origin. This is because planets have to be formed first (the habitat) before life can start and evolution proceed.

It seems that the formation of the universe began when a Big Bang occurred, 13.7 billion years ago, and the universe is still expanding now. Some Kabbalists believe that all souls that were ever created were created then and no more were added.

The Doppler Effect detected is the scientific 'proof' of this on-going expansion ever since. However, before the Big Bang occurred, it is said that matter came from a single point, called the Singularity, which also accommodates space. The whole universe was contained in a point. This huge explosion occurred in a very short span of time – 10 times minus 43 seconds at a point 46.5 billion light years away from us now.

Light travels at 186,000 miles per second or 300,000km per second. At the Big Bang, time, matter and space suddenly existed. The first light of the universe was also formed from the Bang, and is called Cosmic Microwave Background, CMB. The drifting matter formed the inter-stellar clouds and one billion years later, the first stars and galaxies were formed.

The elements generated from the Bang was still limited in type, until a Super Nova was formed, from which heavier elements were created, and thus completing the atoms needed to form matter. About 4.5 billion years ago, our sun condensed from the initial galactic dust and debris. Gravity came into existence and kept the planets in position, rotating round our sun. Our moon was formed from a part of earth after our planet was hit by another planet about 30 to 50 million years after formation of the solar system.

Uranus was also hit by a huge mass, as was Venus, which resulted in an opposite rotation till today. The mysterious Black Holes in the universe were also formed from stars becoming Super Novas, the nearest is about 8,000 light years from us and then Super Novas turn into Black Holes. These can be classified as large, small, and dormant. They generate gamma ray bursts of energy that can potentially wipe out life in the solar system. A Black Hole also consumes everything in its path, even light. Nothing escapes from the intense gravity that it generates. Galactic Black Holes can consume an entire galaxy, while Stellar Black Holes drift across space. Theoretically there are Microscopic Black Holes but these are yet to be discovered. Dormant Holes actually stabilize our galaxy.

Dark Matter makes up 95% of the universe and it can not be seen or measured as yet. Its existence is due to the phenomenon of gravity bending light. Dark Matter keeps the universe together. Dark Energy is the most mysterious phenomena of the entire universe, it being an anti-gravity force that accelerates as the universe expands. Scientists believe that one day, the universe will stop expanding and this is called the Big Freeze, following the 2nd Law of Thermodynamics, where galaxies will just disintegrate and everywhere there will only be Black Holes. The condition of Absolute Zero is reached and all motion stops. Other theories of the end are the Big Rip and Big Crunch.

In the Big Rip, Dark Energy keeps increasing until it is out of control and galaxies will be ripped apart, about 20 billions years from now. The more positive theory is the Big Crunch, giving us more time, say 50 billion years from now, where galaxies collide and merge and then we are back to a single point – Singularity.

The Big Bang Theory has some flaws and to overcome this, it is proposed that the initial explosion was accompanied by a sudden massive expansion in a fraction of a second, followed by a slower one. The Theory of Relativity by Einstein explains very well the physics of galaxy and planets but at an atomic level, Quantum Mechanics is the workable model. However to explain both extremes, these Theories are not able to do so.

Space and time are all distorted in the sub-atomic world. Thus it was proposed the String Theory which explains Gravity, Electromagnetic, Strong and Weak Forces all in one formula. It is thus regarded as a theory of everything. Basically it means that when these forces vibrate differently, it gives different mass and charge. It also predicts there are extra dimensions and these are all around us and these dimensions can be curved or coiled, and referred to as Calabi-Yau shapes.

Witten argues that there should be eleven space time dimensions in all, as demanded by the M Theory. The existence of the extra dimensions accounts for all the mathematical Constants that exist in the field of universal calculations, perfectly. However, the scientists have put themselves in another fix because there are now five versions of String Theory and they all appear equally valid. To me, the grand universe is a mechanism as well as a living organism. I came to this conclusion during one of my meditations.

The above discussions are scientific theories to make us have a sense of the immense universe and cosmos, with all the juicy secrets they hold, and if we project our thoughts outwards, we will see that what a miniscule atom we are, with a similar beginning and ending. We are indeed all One. Therefore, think, act and be as One. Just as Einstein unified space, time and gravity in an equation while others have shown that electromagnetic force and weak nuclear forces are part of one and the same force, the electroweak force.

The above scientifically based descriptions are to show that even in the scientific circles, many prominent scientists believe in a single beginning for all things. That is why they spend a lifetime trying to unify all the theories.

The ancient Chinese unified the forces in the form of 64 hexagrams of the I Ching, The Book of Changes. These were in turn derived from the eight trigrams. And these eight trigrams were derived from the foundation of the philosophy of The Great Primal Beginning, which generates two primary forces, the yin and yang, then the two generate the four images and the four give rise to the eight trigrams. In other words, from one it became two, then four and then eight. Again, it all began with one – The Great Primal Beginning. In unifying some principles, the Chinese stumbled upon the I Ching and its myriad uses to help mankind, such as its great divination powers and also as the basis of Feng Shui. The sage, Lao Tzu, in his Tao Te Ching chapter 40 also hinted of the unity principle and he put it as shown below:–

".....All things come from the Way
And the Way comes from nothing"
How beautiful and profound this statement is.

Suffice to say, we are all given the free will to choose how to perceive every thing and through our perceptions we form the basis of our beliefs.

The Bible introduced us to Adam and Eve, and from them we originated. The anthropologists are still piecing together the beginnings of mankind from archaeological findings. They are getting closer to prove that we all originated from one family, perhaps from Africa. Darwin's theory was that we came from the apes but one Hopi Indian elder said it very nicely that only the Whites believed that our ancestors were from the apes while the Hopi thinks that the apes were our cousins. Even the Cherokee Indian tribe, in their story, had the concept of One, expressed as the 'Three in One" of Sound, Light and Will. The debate goes on.

From the Hindu Isavasya Upanishad, even at the time of before Buddha (500BC), it described very well this concept of being One in another way – 'He who sees all beings in his own self and his own self in all beings does not suffer from any repulsion by that experience.'

It seems we have come full circle and it has become the 'New Age' to say we are all one. Many of us are believers that everything is energy and with this comes no separation, we are all connected.

I think regardless of the real answer, there is enough wisdom in many cultures to put forth the concept of all humanity belonging to the same family.

So what is the great thing about this idea of being One? The answer I have is from Sai Baba himself, to whom I feel a special link. He conveyed that if we can feel and think that we all belong to the same family of souls, then only can we do likewise with the Divine! This is the secret that enables us to be one with the gods.

Sai Baba said that true cognition of God begins only when the flame of your heart becomes a part of the Divine Fire. When we feel we are close to Him to the extent that we behave, think and be like Him, is being one with Him, then He can be with us in our hearts and guide us in our daily lives.

It is believed and proven by scientists, it is thought by modern age thinkers and is written or depicted in every traditional religion in some way or another for instance Jesus said, in John 10:30, 'I and my Father are one.'

Just as our bodies are one whole consciousness and cannot be separated, severed or divided and still be a whole, so it is with everything smaller than us and all things bigger; so it is with the Earth, the Universe and beyond. We Are All One.

23. The Cosmic Man

I have related many experiences in my life while working as a doctor. I have much more to tell but it is not the appropriate time yet. As you can infer, my outlook is different from that of many people. I strive for perfection - the following sentences resonates with me "be you perfect as the Father is perfect".

I try to understand the human body, mind and spirit as well as the Cosmos. This journey itself has taken a huge part of my energy and life, first fighting for a place to study medicine, then doing the various post-graduate courses and then exploring the various metaphysics of life by studying the esoteric sciences.

I have recalled various aspects of my past life, expanded my horizon, have been in contact with men and saints. Above all, I am discovering my Higher Self and am learning to communicate with it. My best journey has been to connect with my inner Self. It is indeed a wise saying that to go within is where you have all the answers rather than to go with-out.

I am living in an environment where there is tremendous pressure of race and religion in every day life. However race, religion, nationality and culture no longer influence me for I see you as a soul. Emotions like jealousy, hatred, anger, greed, envy and actions like physically hurting others, are all in my past. Or at least I know how to deal with them now.

I have conquered the fear of the unknown and fear of death as well. Likewise negative words are no longer in my vocabulary. Doing a good deed or just serving the needs of people makes me the happiest. My prayer is to give thanks for every kind of experience I have - be they positive or negative. Let the Tao flow.

The Yin must meet the Yang and embrace. As I live the Truth, the Truth comes to me whenever I seek it. As taught by my mother, I learn to speak to Nature and one day, my plant spoke to me asking me to water it. In our belief, everything has a soul.

I have learned that the best prayers are not for our own selves but for others. Those with health in jeopardy, I learned how to pray for their recovery. I extend my prayers to all human beings, every animal on Mother Earth, everything in Nature including everyone and everything in all Universes.

It is true; the best thing to do is to be able to give rather than to receive all the time. I love to radiate Light and Love. I feel so happy when I say the mantra "Light I am, Light I am; Light Expand, Expand, Expand!"

I try to be the Cosmic Man – bondless and unlimited freedom in all aspects including from time and space. Liberty from any constraints is really a great feeling. Knowledge, wisdom, love, joy and intelligence are the best gifts, apart from having good health.

Remember that if a thing you do is for the benefit of everyone, then you have the Universe supporting your actions. If you only do things for your own benefit, disregarding others, then you are alone.

Life is for us to enjoy God's creations, to grow and improve our soul standing and to be in service to ourselves and others. When we serve in this way, we are actually doing God's work for, remember we are all one!

May the blessings be.

Bibliography and recommended reading

1. Brandon Bays, *The Journey*, (Simon and Schuster, 2002)
2. Deedre Diemer, *The ABCs of Chakra Therapy*, (Samual Weiser, Inc. 1998)
3. Ho Nee Yong, *East Meets West in Education*, (Pearson Malaysia Sdn Bhd., 2009)
4. Arthur Waley, trans., *Lao Tzu, Tao Te Ching*, (Wordsworth Editions Limited, 1997)
5. Wayne W. Dyer, *Change Your Thoughts Change Your Life - Living the Wisdom of the Tao*, (Hay House. 2007)
6. Louise L. Hay – *You Can Heal Your Life*, (Hay House, 1984)
7. The Dr. Edward Bach Centre, Forward by Judy Howard *The Work of Dr Edward Bach, An introduction and guide to the 38 Flower Remedies*, (Wigmore Publications Ltd., Reprint 1997)
8. Katharina Bless, *Flower Healing Power*, (Silver Dove Books, 2004)
9. Harish Johari, *Energy Centres of Transformation*, (Inner Traditions India, 1987)
10. Judy Jacka, *Meditation, The most natural therapy*, (Geddes and Grosset, 2005)

11. Aileen Yeoh, *Longevity, The Tao of Eating and Healing.* (Times Edition- Marshall Cavendish, 1989)

12. Dr Zhi Gang Sha, *The Power of Soul*, (Atria Books, 2009)

13. Osho, *The Book of Secrets*, (St Martin's Griffin, 1974)

14. *Medical Tribune,* 1-15 April, (2009)

15. S. C. Larsson, N. Orsini, A. Wolk, *Processed meat consumption and stomach cancer risk: a meta-analysis.* J Nat, Aug 2.98(15):1078-1087 refer. (Cancer Inst., 2006)

16. World Cancer Research Fund/American institute for Cancer Research, *Food, Nutrition, Physical Activity, and the Prevention of Cancer. A Global Perspective.* (Washington DC. AICR, 2007)

17. R. M. Van Dam, W. C. Willet, E. B. Rimm, M. J. Stampfer, F. B. Hu. *Dietary fat and meat intake in relation to risk of type 2 diabetes in men*, (American Diabetes Association, 2002)

18. Torkom Saraydarain, *The Science of Meditation*, (TSG Publishing Foundation, Inc, 1993).

19. Mantak Chia and Tao Huang, *Door to All Wonders. Application of the Tao Te Ching.* (Universal Tao Publications, 2002)

20. Dr Hock Chye Yeoh, Chapter 40 of *"Obesity", in Medicine: Facts for the layman.* Ed Dr Lee Yan San, (Malaysian Medical Association, 1999)

RESOURCES

Dr H.C. Yeoh's specially formulated Super Food and Super Fiber and other products. For a full description, please read the chapter on "A guide to supplements that make a difference" in this book.

The Super Food

This product is especially suitable for growing children, weight loss, the elderly, busy executives needing a wholesome quick meal and those, travelling, going camping etc. Adding salt and pepper is all that is required. For a more elaborate preparation, even vegetables and pieces of cooked meat or chicken can be added.

The Super Fiber

The gentle but pleasantly effective action will relieve constipation and so is an excellent detoxification agent. It can also be used for reducing weight and cholesterol levels. A healthy gut is the key to a healthy body.

Both the Super Food and Super Fiber are our original formulations.

Probiotics

All the goodness of a genuine probiotic plus some mountain herbs are available in this formulation from Japan.

Active Greens

This drink has the five most precious ingredients of ashitaba leaves, barley grass, chlorella and spirulina to provide enzymes, vitamins, minerals, trace elements, amino acids, fibers and other micronutrients. It makes the perfect combination.

Other services

Medical feng shui to help resolve serious health issues or for prevention of ill health.

Due to logistic issues, this service is confined to those who I can attend to personally.

Speaking engagements

The following topics which covers a very wide range, can be arranged –

1. Health and medical topics
2. Esoteric Knowledge
3. Health motivation talks

Enquiries can be made to yeohawk@gmail.com